PREVENTION OF CORONARY HEART DISEASE AND STROKE

ff

PREVENTION OF CORONARY HEART DISEASE AND STROKE

A workbook for primary care teams

Julian Tudor Hart MB, BChir(Camb.), FRCP, DCH, FRCGP
General Practitioner, Glyncorrwg Health Centre, West Glamorgan

and

Barbara Stilwell RGN, RHV, BSc
Research Fellow, Nurse Practitioner
Department of General Practice, University of Birmingham *and* Birchfield Medical Centre, Handsworth, Birmingham

with a contribution from

J. A. Muir Gray MD
Community Physician, Oxfordshire Health Authority

faber and faber
LONDON · BOSTON

First published in 1988
by Faber and Faber Limited
3 Queen Square, London WC1N 3AU

Photoset, printed and bound in Great Britain by
Redwood Burn Limited, Trowbridge, Wiltshire

British Library Cataloguing in Publication Data

Hart, J. T.
Prevention of coronary heart disease and
stroke: a workbook for primary care teams.
1. Heart—Diseases—Prevention
I. Title II. Stilwell, B. III. Gray, Muir
616.1′205 RC682

ISBN 0–571–14504–3

CONTENTS

ACKNOWLEDGEMENTS

We extend our thanks to all our colleagues who, by sharing knowledge and giving encouragement, helped in the preparation of this book. Particular thanks are due to our secretaries who typed and retyped the much corrected scripts and produced a clean manuscript for the publisher!

Finally, we thank our families, especially Mary and Jon, who continued to support us during many weekends spent writing.

The illustrations are used by permission of the various authors and publishers to whom our thanks are extended:
Figure 4/1 by permission of the Royal College of General Practitioners.
Figure 4/2 by permission of the WHO and Professor Doll.
Figures 6/1 and 6/2 by permission of Longman Group Ltd (Division M), Edinburgh.
Figure 8/1 by permission of the *Lancet* (included in *Lancet* 1973; **2:** 1407–9).

PREFACE

Originally we were invited to write a book for nurses on management of high blood pressure in general practice and community care. However, we soon became convinced that effective management of high blood pressure must take other major cardiovascular risk factors fully into account at every point, and that the whole primary care team needs to learn together. We therefore expanded our remit to include the within-community management of smoking, obesity, high blood cholesterol, and non-insulin-dependent diabetes, and expanded our target audience to include the whole primary care team, doctors, nurses, office staff, and anyone else with an interest in organised work to prevent stroke and heart attacks in general practice.

It has been difficult to write for readers with such diverse training and experience, but we think their common interest in working more effectively to reduce crippling and premature death makes shared learning possible. We doubt if anyone working in general practice will either know so much that they can't learn more from the material we have put together, or so little that they won't understand its arguments, but it will demand patience from a few and fairly hard work from many.

We expect many readers to read some chapters and not others, but this is not a cookery book. There is no way that preventive work on the necessary scale can be simply added to practice as it is now. Big changes in staffing and organisation are eventually inevitable for any team that follows this path, though we recognise that at some point a start has to be made without additional resources. Much attention has therefore been given to fairly general questions of practice organisation, records, and techniques for nurse-consultations or counselling by non-professionals.

We have also had to write about something which as yet hardly exists. All three of us have personal experience of developing preventive work in general practice, but much is going on in many parts of this country and abroad of which we are unaware, or know too little about to include. It is a pioneering field in which we must be confident enough of our general rightness to run the risk of making some mistakes; we hope they are few, but some there certainly are.

We have not written a cookery book, because for a long time to come all the cooks will have to work out their own recipes to meet local needs with local resources. Though we provide little in the way of set formulas, we hope this book will help primary health workers to think and act more effectively, and perhaps also help some administrators and politicians with an interest in preventive work to create a National Health Service in fact as well as in name.

We have included references where we thought it likely that some readers would want to go to the original material, or where controversial statements required access to the evidence on which they are based. We should like to see much wider use of the published literature by all primary health workers in devising their own local strategies. We shall welcome comments, criticism, and positive suggestions for improvement from all readers, whatever their role in the team.

PART ONE: THE PROBLEM

Chapter 1
THE NATURE OF THE PROBLEM

The causes of stroke and coronary heart disease differ in many ways, but they overlap enough to make their prevention possible as a combined operation.

CORONARY HEART DISEASE

Coronary disease develops in two stages. First, waxy plaques (atheroma) are laid down in the walls of the coronary arteries, aorta, and other large and middling arteries, starting in adolescence and accumulating throughout life. These plaques eventually obstruct the flow of blood to the heart muscle, causing transient pain over the front of the chest, usually provoked by exercise and quickly relieved by rest (angina).

One or more coronary arteries may become completely obstructed by a blood clot at a site of reduced coronary blood flow (coronary thrombosis). The blood supply to an area of heart muscle is then halted, resulting in cell-death after a few minutes (myocardial infarction). This usually causes prolonged pain in the front of the chest, sometimes severe, but often dismissed as 'indigestion'. Roughly 20% of all myocardial infarcts cause little or no pain, and are only recognised by measuring heart muscle enzymes, or by electrocardiographic (ECG) changes which may take several hours to develop; this can happen even in major attacks causing heart failure. Very small areas of infarction may cause death if they involve the conducting system of the heart, producing a disordered ventricular rhythm. This may be minor and transient, or chronic but not necessarily life-threatening as in atrial fibrillation, or it may lead to death within a few minutes, as in ventricular fibrillation and cardiac arrest. Roughly 80% of coronary deaths are from disordered rhythms, often from small infarcts; 20% are due to pump failure, with destruction of a large mass of heart muscle. Deaths from disordered rhythm are preventable by resuscitation if this is available within about 7 minutes, followed by conversion to a normal rhythm by an electric defibrillator, and such people may survive another 20 years or more with little or no disability. On the other hand, people with enough heart damage to cause pump failure usually die, either in the attack or within a few months of recovery.

TREATMENT OF HEART ATTACKS

Deaths from disordered rhythm can theoretically be prevented by intensive care in hospital, but in practice few of them are. Roughly half of all the people who have a first heart attack die within the first 2 hours after the onset of chest pain. Salvage has to reach the patient within 2 hours if it is to be effective for more than a lucky few.

As matters now stand in Britain, there is an average 2-hour delay before patients even send for their general practitioner, another 45 minutes before the GP arrives, and an hour and 45 minutes before patients reach hospital; a total delay of 4.5 hours. By then about 60% of all the deaths which are going to happen within a month of the attack have already occurred.

Delay could be reduced by:

1 Encouraging patients and relatives to call for help more quickly and directly.
2 By training ambulance crews in cardiopulmonary resuscitation (CPR) and equipping them with defibrillators.
3 By training the general public in CPR.

In Seattle, USA, survival after heart attacks rose from 21% when bystander CPR was not available, to 43% when it was.[1]

Mass participation in CPR training is now widespread in the USA and Scandinavia and the new Save a Life campaign in the UK is very welcome.

Whatever we do along these lines (and we should do a lot more), the saving of life will certainly be small, compared with the savings that can result from attacking known causes of coronary heart disease.

IS PREVENTION OF CORONARY HEART DISEASE POSSIBLE?

After 40 years of continuously rising coronary death rates in the USA, male deaths from coronary disease began to level off around 1967. They then began to fall, slowly at first, then more steeply, so that altogether between 1963 and 1976 there was a fall of 27%. In Britain, though deaths began to level off a bit from 1973, there is still no sign of a significant fall.

There is still much doubt about why the fall in the USA and Australia has happened, and why it has failed to happen in Britain, Holland, or Scandinavia, but one thing is certain: coronary heart disease in early middle age is not an inevitable result of a good standard of living. Coronary heart attacks can be prevented without imposing an intolerably spartan lifestyle on the general population. A probable but less certain conclusion is that efforts at community level to control coronary disease in the USA, which stand in such sharp contrast to inactivity in Britain, really have paid off. One does not have to believe everything claimed by American enthusiasts for jogging, vegetarianising, transcendentally meditating, by-pass grafting, and 'zapping' every diastolic pressure above 90mmHg, to admit that they must be doing something right.

In Britain there has been much talk but little action. One reason for this could be that talking is a lot cheaper than doing. It takes time and labour to identify local needs and to explain them to ordinary people in their own language, starting from where they are at, not where some professionals assume they ought to be.

Where health services concentrate on salvage of disease that has already occurred, primary care teams can be small, perhaps just a GP plus a receptionist, backed by the full resources of a hospital. But where responsibility goes back to the beginnings of disease, to anticipatory care and prevention, we need larger teams with wider responsibilities. People will not eat more thoughtfully, use their leisure more vigorously, or accept a lifetime of pill-taking unprompted by symptoms, just because of a 30-second speech from their GP, backed by a leaflet from the stack in the waiting room, and even these are a lot more than most patients get now. Mass re-education demands mass educators, with time for each person in the population at risk, both in groups and in individual consultation. The educators must themselves be educated, and that needs more people again. Studies of diabetics in St Thomas' Hospital in London showed that in order to understand their own management and thus be able to take most of the responsibility for it, patients needed a total of 4 hours organised learning, mostly in small groups or on a one-to-one basis. People at high risk of coronary disease have almost as much to learn, and to change about how they live, as diabetics. This learning will not happen unless primary care teams have enough staff, appropriately trained, and with enough time to make room for these new tasks against the competing priorities of helping people who are already sick.

RISK FACTORS FOR CORONARY HEART DISEASE

Coronary disease causing angina has been common in Britain for at least 2 centuries, but complete obstruction of coronary arteries by blood clot (coronary thrombosis, myocardial infarction), and sudden death from disordered heart rhythm which seems to be closely related to this, seem to have been rare before the First World War, and became common only in the early 1930s.

Studies of whole populations since the Second World War, at first mainly in the USA but now repeated in most parts of Europe, have defined risk factors measurable in individuals which predict subsequent coronary events in groups. It is possible for individuals to survive without coronary events despite the presence of these risk factors, just as some will survive even if they cross the road with their eyes shut and their fingers stuffed in their ears. The following 9 risk factors are now established by consistent evidence from large population surveys in many parts of the developed world:

1	male	**SEX**
2		**F**amily History
3		**A**ge
4		**G**lucose Intolerance (Diabetes)
5		**S**moking
6	blood	**C**holesterol
7		**O**besity
8	blood	**P**ressure
9		**S**loth (life without physical exertion).

These, you may have noticed, form the mnemonic 'SEX FAGS COPS'. Whether true or not, it is at least memorable.

Two known groups of risk factors are missing from this list: those associated with *personality*, and those associated with *race* and *social class*. These are difficult to measure, and theories about them are difficult to disprove (and therefore to prove in a scientific way). They show big differences between countries so that it may be misleading to apply research done in the USA or Britain to other parts of the world, but there does appear to be a high rate of heart disease in people from the Indian subcontinent. Throughout the developed countries, poor people get more early coronary disease than rich people, but in economically undeveloped countries, the rich get much more coronary disease than the poor. Some but certainly not all of these differences arise from differences in the nine classical risk factors listed, particularly smoking and obesity.

Even when all known risk factors are taken into account, many heart attacks happen in fairly young people, which are not predictable from these known risks. It now seems likely that many of these are connected with changes in *blood clotting*, which may precede a heart attack by only two or three years.

STROKE

A stroke is a loss of brain substance, revealed by impairment of brain function for 24 hours or more, caused by interruption of arterial blood supply to the brain. Losses of function lasting less than 24 hours, also caused by interruptions of arterial blood supply, are called transient ischaemic attacks (TIAs). They are closely related to strokes, they indicate an exceptionally high risk of stroke, and methods of preventing them are almost the same. Between a quarter and one-third of all strokes are quickly fatal. Of people who survive, from half to three-quarters eventually walk and are able to live more or less independently. The rest either become dependent on their families, if they have them, or end their days in institutional care.

First strokes are usually much less disabling than later ones, and may be a useful warning that preventive action, usually control of high blood pressure, is urgent. Many transient episodes, which at first appear to have cleared up completely within 24 hours and to be classifiable as TIAs, can be shown to have caused some permanent loss of brain function, by taking a really careful history from friends and relatives, by applying formal tests of brain function (such as subtracting 7s from 100, or recalling the day's events confirmed by someone from the family), and (least importantly) by a careful search for physical signs of central nervous system (CNS) damage. True TIA's are caused by small platelet emboli originating in the carotid or vertebrobasilar arteries, and usually last only a few minutes.

True strokes are of three kinds: embolic, thrombotic, and haemorrhagic.

Embolic strokes are caused by clots of arterial blood, detached usually from a fibrillating left atrium in heart failure, or from the lining of an atheromatous carotid artery. The clot lodges in a brain artery, causing infarction of brain tissue in the same way that coronary thrombosis causes infarction of heart muscle. Evidence of severe carotid atheroma (a murmur or reduced pulsation) on either side of the neck (not necessarily on the same side as the brain damage), or evidence of atrial fibrillation, together with a sudden onset, all point towards a diagnosis of embolic stroke.

Thrombotic strokes usually start more slowly, often during the night so that the patient is first found to have some paralysis and/or speech impairment on waking up. They are caused by clotting of arterial blood in a brain artery narrowed by atheroma.

Thrombotic and embolic strokes together account for about 80% of all strokes, and about 15% of these are associated with atrial fibrillation, mostly from coronary heart disease and/or high blood pressure, but some of it from thyrotoxic heart disease (often apparent only from thyroid function tests) or rheumatic valvular disease. The other 20% of strokes are caused by bleeding (haemorrhage).

Haemorrhagic strokes are usually severe, usually cause severe headache (if the patient is conscious), and are often impossible to distinguish from thrombotic or embolic strokes, unless facilities for computerised axial tomography (CAT scan) are available. Intracerebral haemorrhage occurs at weak points in the brain arteries called *Microaneurysms* (Charcot–Bouchard aneurysms), small blebs in the arterial walls, usually numerous and mainly caused by high blood pressure. Subarachnoid haemorrhage is usually easily recognised and distinguished from other causes of stroke by its sudden onset with severe headache, neck stiffness, and vomiting. Subarachnoid haemorrhage occurs from bursting of *berry aneurysms*. These are much larger, about the size of a pea, often present from childhood, and are not caused by high blood pressure, though they are more likely to burst if pressure is high.

Treatment of strokes

Whereas the heart can usually make a fair functional recovery from all but the largest infarcts (the ones that cause pump failure), the different parts of the brain are too specialised for this, and most brain damage is permanent. Little can be done for people who have had strokes except: (1) to give excellent nursing care, sometimes more readily available from community nurses than in understaffed geriatric wards; (2) to be reasonably sure that it really is a vascular stroke, rather than a rare but more treatable disorder such as a subdural haematoma, brain abscess, or operable brain tumour; and (3) to use all available family and community resources to support re-entry into as active a life as possible.

In general, the sad truth is that treatment has much less to offer stroke victims than coronary victims. Prevention of stroke, on the other hand, is much easier and better understood than prevention of coronary heart disease. When strokes do happen, it is worth while for the whole primary care team to review the patient's record to see whether this risk could have been anticipated and avoiding action taken. Strokes in people with blood pressures at or over 175/105mmHg can be reduced by about half by controlling high blood pressure, which amounts to about 15% of all strokes. Some others can be prevented by using long-term anticoagulants in atrial fibrillation.

RISK FACTORS FOR STROKE

These differ from the risk factors for coronary heart disease.

Way out in front as a cause of all forms of stroke (thrombotic, haemorrhagic, or embolic) is high blood pressure, which accounts for about two-thirds of the known causal factors operating. More important, it is a reversible cause. Though there is still no convincing controlled evidence that reduction of high blood pressure prevents coronary heart attacks, there is overwhelming evidence that treatment is effective in preventing strokes.

The second major cause is heart failure, particularly if this is accompanied by atrial fibrillation. Accurate, regularly supervised treatment of heart failure with digoxin, diuretics, and sometimes vasodilators almost certainly reduces stroke risk. Heart failure itself can often be prevented by treating high blood pressure.

The third major contributor to stroke is age. Risk of stroke rises rapidly from about 45 years. In general, peak ages for strokes are about 10 years later than peak ages for coronary heart attacks, in all populations.

Other causal factors lag way behind these three in importance. High blood viscosity (packed cell volume (PCV) >0.45) roughly doubles stroke risk, and reduction by monthly venesection may be worth while at very high PCVs, say 0.50+, but there is still no controlled evidence on this. Diabetes increases stroke risk by two or three times, and accurate control of diabetes, desirable for many other reasons, may help to reduce this risk.

Unlike coronary risk, stroke risk seems not to be affected much by cigarette smoking or blood cholesterol, though obesity seems to be fairly important, and heavy alcohol drinking very important. Again, there are other and better reasons why people of all ages should not smoke.

CONCLUSION

Prevention of coronary heart attacks and strokes depends on control of their causes. Risk factors (predictive measurements) are not necessarily causes, so reducing the risk factors does not always reduce risk. On present evidence, stopping smoking and even fairly small reductions in blood cholesterol seem to be very effective in reducing risk of coronary heart attacks. There is no convincing evidence that control of high blood pressure has much effect on risk of coronary heart attacks, but it is very effective in preventing stroke and heart failure.

These arguments apply to reduction of risk in people who have not yet had a heart attack or stroke (primary prevention). Prevention of subsequent attacks, in people who have already had one (secondary prevention), is a somewhat different problem, considered in detail in Chapter 8.

REFERENCE

1 Thompson GR, Hallstrom AP, Cobb LA. Bystander-initiated cardiopulmonary resuscitation in the management of ventricular fibrillation. *Annals of Internal Medicine* 1979; **90**:737.

Chapter 2
THE SIZE OF THE PROBLEM

HOW MANY FATAL HEART ATTACKS AND STROKES?

In men aged 45–54, more than half of all deaths are caused by coronary heart disease, stroke, or other closely related arterial disease. This is twice the number dying from cancers, and more than seven times the number dying from accidents. Figures for women in the same age-group are about half those for men.

The average GP with a list of about 2000 of all ages, will have 8 fatal and 13 non-fatal coronary heart cases a year, and 3 fatal and 4 non-fatal stroke cases.

Where do they happen?

There are big regional differences in Britain, with high stroke and coronary rates in Northwest Scotland, the North of England, and Wales, and low rates in East Anglia and the South-east.

In general, these geographical differences fit in with the known distribution of major risk factors. Even more, they fit into the distribution of coronary deaths by social class. Figure 2/1 shows the difference between observed and expected deaths from diseases of the circulatory system (nearly all of it coronary heart disease) by social class for men aged 15–64 in 1970–72 (the latest years available). 3500 fewer men in social classes I and II (professional and managerial) and 8302 more men in social

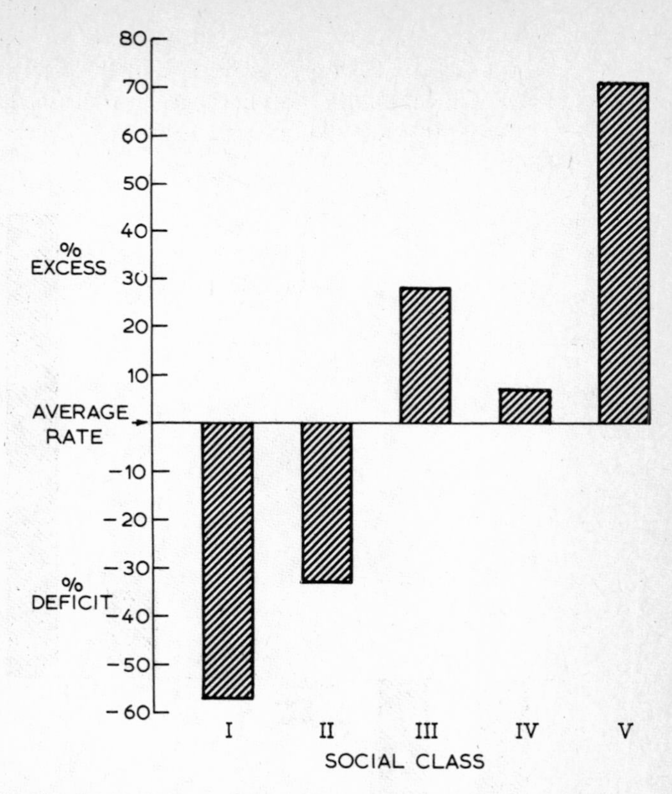

Fig. 2/1 Ratio of observed to expected deaths from ischaemic heart disease by social class, men aged 35–44, 1970–72 (OPC, 1978[1])

classes III, IV and V (clerical, skilled, semi-skilled and unskilled manual workers) died from coronary disease under 65 than would have been expected if coronary death rates were the same in all social classes. Social class differences are greatest in younger men. For the youngest age-group with a significant number of deaths, 35–44, death rates for unskilled labourers were 65% above the average for all men, whereas men in the professional and managerial classes had death rates 54% below it.

Even more striking are the social class differences for stroke (Fig. 2/2). Unskilled labourers aged 35–44 were more than twice as likely to die of cerebrovascular disease as the average for all men, whereas professional and managerial men in that age-group were about 50% less likely to die from this cause.

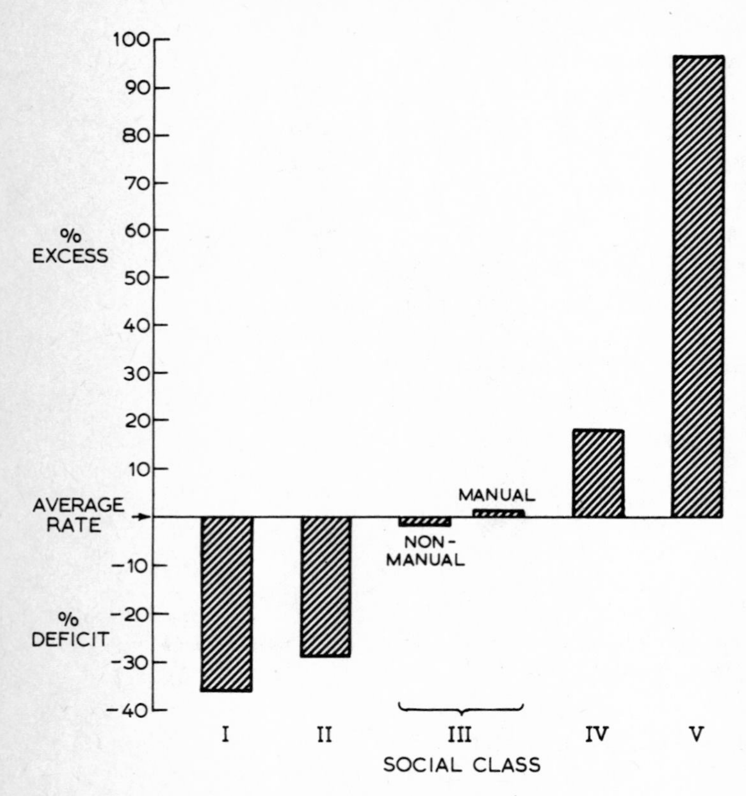

Fig. 2/2 Social class differences for stroke (OPC, 1978[1])

These social differences mean that some local populations have a much bigger problem than others. In general, poor communities, with the biggest burdens of disease and most difficult problems of prevention, have the least resources to deal with them (the Inverse Care Law).[2] For primary care teams serving mixed populations, more work is required to make information about prevention understandable and acceptable to manual workers than to white collar workers and the managerial class.

HOW MANY HYPERTENSIVES?

Between 7 and 10% of the British population aged 35–64 have diastolic pressures >100mmHg (phase 5: disappearance of sound), or systolic pressures >170mmHg. On the evidence of controlled trials all these people need antihypertensive treatment of some kind, not necessarily antihypertensive drugs, and those with diastolic pressures averaging 110mmHg or more (about 4% of the population in this age-group) certainly need medication.

Another 15–20% have diastolic pressures >90mmHg, or systolic pressures >150mmHg. These borderline hypertensives are not, on present controlled evidence, likely to gain more than they will lose by starting treatment with antihypertensive drugs, unless they have evidence of organ damage, but they do need systematic follow-up once a year.

To this caseload we must add people over 65, who began treatment in middle age and should continue; and those elderly hypertensives who develop signs of organ damage, or who develop systolic pressures averaging >180mmHg.

Altogether, a practice population of 2000 (all ages) should expect to have to care for 130–150 people on antihypertensive drugs. Another 150–200 borderline or elderly untreated hypertensives will need to be followed up at least once a year. Many of these are likely to need treatment in the future and are at relatively high risk.

WHO WILL LOOK AFTER THEM?

The preventive health care of millions of people has been left to the initiative of a few enthusiasts, with usually untrained and understaffed teams, groping their way forward without serious planning or support either locally or nationally from the machinery of the National Health Service (NHS). The result is that even the most obviously necessary work is not being done. Representative samples of GP-registered populations show that only 30–40% of all men over 20 have ever had their BP noted in their GP records (charts) over a 10-year period.[3,4] Inner-city practice is even worse, with BP recorded in only 4–22%.[5,6] Even very high and very dangerous pressures, say 220/150mmHg, can and often do persist for months or years without symptoms, finally presenting with stroke or heart failure. Where all BPs are not measured, all severe hypertension cannot be identified and treated. Even when hypertension is recognised, quality of assessment and follow-up is often poor. From a third to a half of hypertensives are started on treatment after only 1 BP reading, less than 1 in 20 have their urine tested for glucose and protein, and about a third of those started on treatment are lost to follow-up. The preventive work could be done by many more primary care teams, however, and this book will tell you how.

HOW MANY SMOKERS?

If up to 10% of adults with moderate to severely raised blood pressure overload the system, what can we expect from the average 42% of the adult population who smoke?

People rarely consult a GP about smoking, but about 20% of all GP consultations are about its most obvious consequence, middle and lower respiratory tract disease. In how many of these is there even an enquiry about smoking? Though two-thirds of one group of GP trainers claimed that they routinely recorded smoking habits in all their patients' records, audit of a random sample of those records (by the same GPs) showed that less than a third of the records actually contained any reference to smoking habits.[7]

Yet smoking causes 90% of deaths from lung cancer (now the commonest site of cancer in men and second only to breast cancer in women), 75% of deaths from chronic bronchitis, and at least 25% of all coronary deaths in men under 65; between 50 000 and 100 000 deaths each year in Britain. Surveys have shown that 70% of smokers say they want to stop, but only 10%

can recall any doctor ever having specifically advised them to do so.

HOW MANY PEOPLE WITH OBESITY OR DIABETES?

These two problems are interconnected, because obese people are more likely to develop diabetes, and both obesity itself and diabetes are risk factors for coronary disease and stroke (though diabetes is a much bigger risk than obesity alone).

Obesity can be conveniently measured as Body Mass Index (BMI, also known as Quetelet's Index), which is:

$$\frac{\text{weight in kilograms (kg)}}{\text{height in metres square (m}^2\text{)}}$$

The upper limit of normal for BMI is conventionally defined as 25.0, but obesity shortens life substantially from about BMI 30.0, so in this book we have defined medical obesity as BMI 30+.

Why do people with BMI 30+ die early? Because around this level, obesity begins to cause, first, glucose intolerance, and then frank diabetes, raised blood pressure and reduced exercise. All these are risk factors for coronary disease, and some are also risk factors for stroke.

Roughly 12% of the middle-aged working-class population are obese by this definition, less in a middle-class population. As matters now stand, few get any systematic help from their GPs or anyone else in the primary care team. About 2% of all adults are frank diabetics, with very high risks of coronary disease and stroke. Most of them have an obesity problem. Nowadays, diabetics rarely die of diabetes; they die of its complications, which occur more often in those with poor control of blood glucose, above all those with poor dietary control. Even known diabetics often have little or no effective medical supervision. One study of a GP population of 20 000 showed that about a quarter of known diabetics had regular supervision from their GP, another quarter had regular supervision from a hospital outpatient department, and the remaining half had no medical supervision at all, just repeat prescriptions from a receptionist.[8]

HOW MANY WITH HIGH BLOOD CHOLESTEROL?

This is a more difficult question to answer. How high is 'high'? Unfortunately the definition of 'normal' puts at least two-thirds of any adult British population into the 'abnormal' high blood cholesterol category. Numbers like this cannot be handled on a mainly individual basis, above all because eating customs generally are shared in families and socially. A mass-education approach is essential. GPs have hitherto generally assumed that their responsibilities begin and end with the individual consultation, perhaps expanded to include preventive advice. To be effective in this kind of prevention, the primary care team will have to learn to play a part in initiating and maintaining the activity of local groups in their own neighbourhoods, reinforcing national health education through the mass media by translation into local speech and custom, in terms of the real choices open to real people.

COMBINED RISKS

In real life, risk factors can't be isolated. High blood pressure, smoking, obesity, high blood cholesterol and diabetes don't exist on their own as diseases: they are distortions of normal physiology usually occurring more than one at a time.

The separate and variously combined effects of the three biggest risk factors have been studied in several large surveys in the USA, whose results were combined in the Pooling Project.[9] Defining the risk factors as:

1 total blood cholesterol > 6.5mmol (250mg)/dl
2 diastolic BP > 90mmHg
3 any current use of cigarettes

the Pooling Project found a steep rise in risk of coronary events for men with all three risk factors, compared with those with any two, any one, or none at all.

Only 17% of the adult population aged 30–59 have none of these risks, so our combined target groups include 83% of the people in this age-band in the average practice. If we were to concentrate our efforts only on the 8% with all three risks, we should be ignoring four-fifths of all coronary events that will occur in the other risk groups. There seems to be no real alternative to tackling the entire middle-aged population, starting at age 30.

For people with more than one major risk factor, subtraction of any one of them may have a disproportionately large effect in reducing risk. This is particularly important for smokers because for coronary disease, at least, smoking is usually in the long run an easier risk to remove than either high blood cholesterol or high blood pressure, and the benefits of stopping extend to prevention of lung and some other cancers and airways obstruction as well as coronary disease.

HIGH AND LOW RISK STRATEGIES

It is a serious and unfortunately frequent error to pose the high risk and the mass approach as alternatives from which we must choose. It is absurd to devise plans only to deal with very high risk groups while ignoring the population within which they live, if only because behaviour is usually determined by groups more than by individuals, by collective fashion more than by personal choice, though we like to see ourselves otherwise. Jogging is unthinkable for most people until lots of other people are doing it, so are wholemeal bread and semi-skimmed milk, or not smoking in a pub. Equally it is absurd for primary health workers, nurses and doctors experienced in helping sick people, to turn away from those in most urgent need of help, and apply themselves only to mass education of which they have no experience at all. Excessive zeal in either direction is likely to lead many GPs and nurses to opt out altogether, becoming cynical about the anticipatory care of the high risk cases, and leaving preventive work for the rest of the local population to be done by other more suitable people, which really means nobody.

A PRACTICAL MODEL FOR RISK SCORING

A practical model for risk scoring in general practice has been developed and used in screening 40 000 people aged 20–59 at 19 health centres in the United Kingdom.[10] This scoring system is derived from the US Pooling Project and the Framingham Project and may not be ideal for a British population, but until we have more results from the British Regional Heart Study and the WHO MONICA project, there is no alternative. The model has been developed in and is designed for large health centres, with a room set aside for a specially trained nurse, with a combination of opportunist screening during ordinary consultations or other contacts with health centre staff (50%), self-referral by patients alerted by local publicity (16%) or recruited by relatives or friends who have already been screened (34%).

During a 10-minute interview the purpose of screening is explained and the following data collected: smoking habit, alcohol intake, family history, education, occupation, presence of corneal arcus or xanthomas, blood pressure, weight, height, and blood total cholesterol concentration. Results are immediately available for discussion with patients because cholesterol is measured by an automated technique (Reflotron, Boehringer Corporation) using capillary blood, and all data are used to calculate a risk score using a 10 megabyte Apricot xi computer. The authors give no data on the time taken to explain the results and give advice and recommendations, but the 19 health centres between them have been able to process 1600 patients a week.

Unlike many previous projects, this model seems to have been very successful in reaching men (44%) almost as well as women, and in avoiding preferential recruitment of middle-class people (20% of those screened were unemployed and 50% had left school without any qualifications). It was less successful in reaching young people, and smokers were probably under-represented – (69% of screenees were non-smokers). The only major risk missing from this formula is glucose intolerance. Diabetics have roughly twice the risk of non-diabetics, other things being equal. Excellent control (HbA1c (see p. 182) maintained at 8% or less) probably eliminates this risk.

This simple formula hardly seems to require a computer, and it seems to us that it could be put to effective use by any primary health worker in all circumstances, whether it be one doctor and one nurse in a single-handed practice, or a giant patient-factory of the type described in the original report. Wherever it is used, its advantage is that it can help both health workers and patients to understand that effective action can be taken on any risk factor or combination of risk factors, with a calculable effect on overall risk, and that it is absurd to act on one risk, such as high blood pressure, while ignoring another, such as smoking.

The authors claim that the model was acceptable to health centre personnel, but no evidence is given about how this conclusion was reached. Discussion with one nurse who worked on this project (who may of course have been atypical) revealed serious problems of job dissatisfaction. She had no opportunity to follow up her patients to see the results of her work, and she found the rapid, highly structured, almost industrialised nature of the work very unrewarding. As large health centres tend easily to slide into impersonal and, therefore, ultimately ineffective styles of care, her experience seems ominous. The model as published is probably good for detection, but will it give good long-term results in changed patient-behaviour?

CONCLUSION

The work required for coronary and stroke prevention in primary care is on a much larger scale than anything previously undertaken by GPs. Only 17% of the middle-aged adult population is free from known risk factors as conventionally defined. Action is necessary on combined rather than single risks, and routine use of a risk-score formula is an important step towards this approach, which we strongly recommend. The task will be much greater in poor districts than rich ones, but even in the best social circumstances, more investment in staff and in-service training will be needed. Present efforts are only on a token scale, but are important as pioneering models for what must be a much bigger undertaking in the near future.

REFERENCES

1 Office of Population and Census Studies. *Occupational mortality: the Registrar General's decennial supplement for England and Wales*, 1970–72, series DS No. 1. London: HMSO, 1978.
2 Hart JT. The Inverse Care Law. *Lancet* 1971; **1**: 405.
3 Ritchie LD, Currie AM. Blood pressure recording by general practitioners in northeast Scotland. *British Medical Journal* 1983;**286**:107.
4 Lawrence MS. Hypertension in general practice. *British Medical Journal* 1984;**288**:1156.
5 Kurji KH, Haines AP. Detection and management of hypertension in general practices in northwest London. *British Medical Journal* 1984;**288**:903.
6 Michael G. Quality of care in managing hypertension by case-finding in northwest London. *British Medical Journal* 1984;**288**:906.
7 Fleming DM, Lawrence MSTA. An evaluation of recorded information about preventive measures in 38 practices. *Journal of the Royal College of General Practitioners* 1981;**31**:615.
8 Doney BJ. An audit of the care of diabetics in a group practice. *Journal of the Royal College of General Practitioners* 1976;**26**:734.
9 Pooling Project research group. Relationship of blood pressure, serum cholesterol, smoking habit, relative weight and ECG abnormalities to incidence of major coronary events. Final report. *Journal of Chronic Diseases* 1978;**31**:201–301.
10 Anggard EE, Land JM, Lenihan CJ et al. Prevention of cardiovascular disease in general practice: a proposed model. *British Medical Journal* 1986;**293**:177.

PART TWO: WHAT CAN BE DONE ABOUT IT?

Chapter 3 AGE, SEX AND FAMILY HISTORY

What can be done about these as risk factors? About them, obviously nothing; with them, quite a lot.

AGE AS A RISK FACTOR

Age is the most powerful of all risks. The older you are, the more likely you are to die not only from coronary disease or stroke, but from almost any cause.

You have to die of something; why not of a sudden fatal stroke or heart attack? Providing the end is swift, complete, and well into an otherwise healthy old age, few of us would prefer any other way. Most old people are rightly mistrustful of therapeutic enthusiasm, and think it would be better directed at the young or middle-aged, who have not already proved their ability to survive.

For prevention, the greatest benefit is to be gained by concentrating effort on younger people, but this alone does not justify the decision. Much more important is the generally convincing evidence that reduction of most risk factors is less effective in the elderly than in middle age, particularly in preventing coronary disease. The evidence for stroke prevention is rather different.

At what age should we stop organised searching?

The major known risk factors do not apply to the elderly as they do to the young and middle-aged. In so far as we know about this at all (there has been much less research in this age-group), the risk factors are less predictive, and generally their control has less effect on stroke, and much less effect on coronary heart disease. These remarks apply particularly to control of smoking and blood cholesterol, less so to control of blood pressure.

The moral is (for coronary disease, at least), that if we are going to do anything to prevent premature deaths, we have to start before the process of coronary atheroma becomes complete and irreversible; probably before 50, certainly before 65.

For prevention of stroke and heart failure, the case is different, but not much. Strokes are caused not only by atheroma in the arteries within and leading to the brain, but by the bursting of microaneurysms, and emboli associated with heart failure. Heart failure itself is commonly (in Britain, probably most commonly) caused by years of overwork for the heart muscle in maintaining high blood pressure. High blood pressure, therefore, continues to be an important and reversible cause of stroke and heart failure, long after it has ceased to be a reversible cause of coronary heart attacks.

However, this should probably have little effect on the age-definition of our target population for prevention. So long as we include everyone up to 65, few new cases of severe hypertension (systolic BP >200mmHg) will appear in old people, if their BP was not already raised (BP >170/100mmHg) between 60–64. There is still no controlled evidence which justifies starting antihypertensive drug treatment for moderate hypertension in the elderly, unless they have evidence of organ damage.

Age-limits for planned prevention

We therefore suggest an upper age-limit of 65 for planned prevention of coronary disease and stroke in whole practice populations. Of course, this is a general strategy; it doesn't mean that we shouldn't do our best to anticipate and if possible avoid cardiovascular disease, particularly heart failure and stroke, in our elderly patients, or that we shouldn't improve the care we give them now. What it does mean is that we should aim our general cardiovascular prevention package at people of working age.

For women, the logical time to start is with first contraceptive advice, usually between 16 and 18, because 3-monthly monitoring of blood pressure and sustained advice on smoking are essential for safe oral contraception.

For men, it is probably best to start at 20, when growth is more or less complete, and it becomes easier to monitor obesity.

Many teams, rightly worried about workload, may want to start later than this in men. The pick-up rate for high blood pressure in men begins to be appreciable at 30–34; starting at 40, as many do, misses out many men at exceptional risk.

SEX AS A RISK FACTOR

Of course, we mean gender. The difference between men and women in death rates for coronary heart attacks is so great that one leading American actuary said it appeared 'almost as if women were a different species'. This is because men are about 6 times as likely to die as women from a coronary heart attack between 35 and 50, but the difference narrows with increasing age, and, in the very old, men are at only slightly higher risk than women. Where there is a high prevalence of coronary disease (for example Britain, USA, and in white South Africans), there is a big difference in risk between men and women; where coronary disease is uncommon or rare (for example Italy, Japan, and in black South Africans), the sex difference is small.

The difference in death rates corresponds to a difference in the prevalence of arterial atheroma found in representative post-mortem material.

There is a wealth of evidence that women are tougher and longer-lived than men, so it is not altogether surprising that a disease like coronary atheroma and thrombosis, which behaves in many ways as a kind of accelerated ageing of the coronary arteries, should happen sooner and more easily in men than in women. Blood pressure, which rises with age in industrialised populations, rises sooner (on average) in men than in women, but this doesn't seem to be an important cause of the sex difference, because even if we compare men and women with the same high levels of blood pressure, the risk of coronary heart attacks is much higher in men than in women. Blood cholesterol levels are generally a little higher in men than in women before the menopause, but after this the average blood cholesterol becomes the same in both sexes. Until the 1970s women mostly smoked much less than men, and part of the past immunity of women from coronary disease must be due to this. Recruitment to smoking is probably the reason that coronary heart death rates for women have been rising in most European countries for the past 20 years or so.

All that refers to coronary disease. It does not apply at all to prevention of stroke and heart failure, to which women are just as prone as men; in fact, a little more, since the men who die young with coronaries do not survive to go into heart failure or have strokes. More women have strokes and heart failure than men, but this just seems to be because they live longer and there are therefore more of them at risk.

More important than all of this is the elementary fact that in most communities, men and women live different lives, work within different social groups, are motivated by different hopes and fears, and therefore require a different approach to prevention, particularly when we are considering group work. The main opinion-formers, the people most willing to innovate and act rather than just talk, are usually women, particularly women with children. Regardless of their personal risk status, if you win the interest and support of this group, you are on the way to shifting community behaviour. All women between 16 and 64 should be included in your target group.

FAMILY HISTORY AS A RISK FACTOR

Family history as a risk factor is powerfully predictive both for stroke and coronary heart disease. Where both parents have a history of coronary disease before retirement age, risk of coronary disease in sons is increased more than five times. If only one parent was affected, risk for sons is doubled. A man who is brother to a man with coronary disease in middle age has three-and-a-half times the risk of one without affected brothers, and a sister in the same position has more than nine times the risk of a sister without affected brothers. Of course, all these refer to coronary disease in middle age or youth; a history of coronary death after normal retirement age doesn't mean much.

These increased risks are partly genetic and partly because families tend to have the same lifestyles. For our practical purposes, the distinction hardly matters.

People can't change their parents, so why does family history matter? In a few cases, certainly less than 1% of all fatal coronary disease, it matters because it can lead to diagnosis of familial hypercholesterolaemia, discussed in Chapter 6. But the real value of collecting systematic family history from the whole target popoulation is that family history is one of the keys to personalising advice and motivating patients to accept necessary changes in lifestyle. Untimely death in parents, brothers or sisters, can be made a powerful means to understanding, providing the experience is discussed with a well-informed doctor or nurse. If it is not discussed, it may be an equally powerful motive for denial either that there is an increased risk or, more commonly, that anything can be done to avert it.

CONCLUSION

The target population for planned prevention of coronary heart disease and stroke, starting from where we are now with the evidence we have, is women from 16 to 64, and men from 20 to 64; if staff time is short, you could make do by starting the men at 30.

Most of the effects of risk factors on coronary heart disease are more or less complete and irreversible by age 50, at least in men, so efforts to reverse them need to be concentrated on people younger than this. Between 50 and 64, the main yield from preventive effort is probably prevention of stroke and hypertensive heart failure rather than coronary heart attacks. By normal retirement age at 65, the whole practice population should have been screened and treated, so that nearly all the people who will ever need antihypertensive drugs should already be on them.

Women are more resistant to coronary disease than men,

and tend to get it about 10 years later. There is no difference between men and women in their liability to stroke and heart failure.

A family history of early coronary disease or stroke is a powerful adverse risk. Knowledge of family history is important in making advice relevant to individual people, and in motivating them to follow it.

Chapter 4
SMOKING

We have to consider what improvements in health might be achieved if smoking were controlled; whether control of smoking is possible; and, if so, how much of this could be done by the primary care team.

WHAT COULD CONTROL OF CIGARETTE SMOKING ACHIEVE?

Cigarette smoking causes at least 50 000 premature deaths each year, 30 000 of them under 65. In 1985 it was calculated that 108 000 people a year are admitted to hospital for smoking-related diseases, using 1 463 000 bed-days at a cost of £111,325,000, according to the British Medical Association (BMA) and the Health Education Council (HEC).

British doctors reduced their average cigarette smoking by two-thirds between 1951 and 1971, whereas there was little change in the smoking habits of the general male population over that time. Doctors' death rates from smoking-related diseases fell by 26%, so their death rate from all causes fell more than three times more than the rate for all men.

SMOKING AND ARTERIAL DISEASE

Smoking is only one of the known causes of coronary disease, but in men under 45 it seems to be the most important, and certainly the most easily reversible.

The effects of cigarette smoking on coronary disease are complex, involving the actions of both nicotine and carbon monoxide, but probably not the tar fraction of tobacco smoke (which is probably the main cause of lung cancer and chronic airways obstruction). These have a long-term effect on the build-up of atheroma in the coronary artery walls, the aorta, and the large arteries to the brain and legs, and probably a short-term effect on the stability of heart rhythm. Figure 4/1 shows the effect of stopping smoking after a first infarct on subsequent coronary death rates.[1]

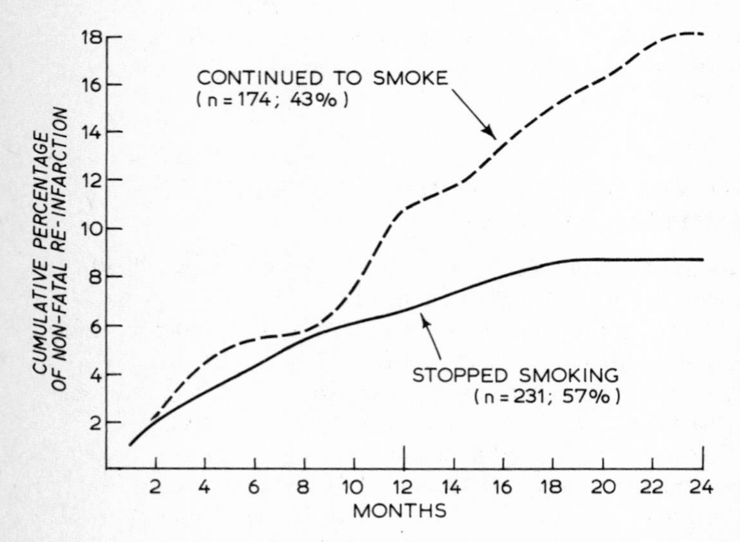

Fig. 4/1 Cumulative percentage of non-fatal relapses following myocardial infarction in 405 patients. Continuing smokers compared with those who stopped[1] (*reproduced by permission RCP*)

There is a rapid fall by almost 50% in the first year (probably because of a reduced risk of ventricular fibrillation and sudden death), followed by a slow decline over the next 20 years to almost the same risk as in lifelong non-smokers (probably because of slower build-up of atheroma). Most of this benefit is to people under 50. Over 65 there is little association between smoking and coronary disease.

Smoking is even more closely associated with peripheral and aortic atheroma than it is with coronary disease. Death from ruptured aortic aneurysm is 6 times commoner in smokers than in non-smokers, and in those smoking 25 or more cigarettes a day it is 10 times commoner. Its effect on atheroma is greatest of all in diabetics, in whom not smoking is as important as the control of diabetes, at least in non-insulin dependent diabetics.

The association of smoking with stroke seems to be small, and smokers who have managed to reach 70 without either angina or peripheral arterial disease should probably be left alone.

SMOKING AND RESPIRATORY DISEASE

Smoking is the most important cause of lung failure from chronic bronchitis and emphysema, and seriously worsens the outlook for asthmatics. Now that rheumatic heart disease is disappearing in industrialised countries, these are now the main cause of heart failure together with high blood pressure and coronary disease. Unlike coronary disease, chronic lung failure, with or without right heart failure (cor pulmonale), seldom shortens life by more than a couple of years, but the impairment of life is appalling. Suffering during the last 3 or 4 years before death in terminal lung failure is often worse than the shorter terminal illness of most cancers.

Examples abound in most industrial working-class communities. They can be a powerful incentive to stop smoking. It is important not to promise too much; lung function rarely improves much once there is significant airways obstruction (peak expiratory flow rate (PEFR) reduced more than 25% below predicted value for sex, height, and age), but as a rule it does stop getting worse.

It is now certain that cigarette smoke from adults has a harmful effect on lung function in children, as well as making it more likely that they will start smoking when they are older.

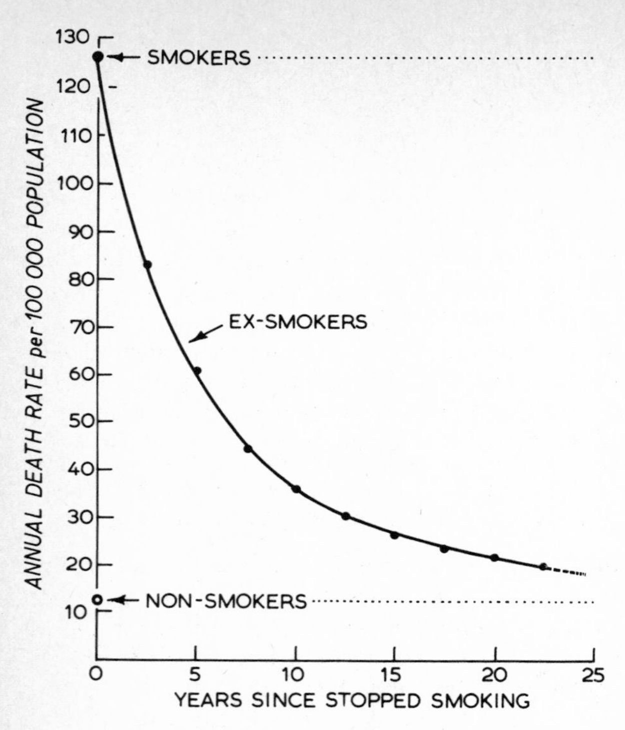

Fig. 4/2 Standardised death rates from lung cancer for cigarette smokers, ex-smokers for various periods and non-smokers (*reproduced by permission of WHO*[2] *and Doll and Hill*[3])

SMOKING AND CANCERS

At least 90% of all lung cancers are caused by cigarette smoking. Lung cancer causes 40% of all cancer deaths in men, in whom it is the commonest site for cancer, and it causes 11% of all cancer deaths in women, in whom it is now the second commonest site for cancer (the breast being the commonest). Because they are smoking less, lung cancer death rates in men have been falling for the past 10 years or so, but lung cancer death rates in women are still rising rapidly, reflecting their continued recruitment to smoking during and since the Second World War. Stopping smoking slowly reduces this risk (Fig. 4/2).[2]

Between 1954 and 1971, the proportion of doctors who smoked cigarettes fell by 50%. Over the same period, their death rate from lung cancer fell by 40%. The rate for the whole male population remained the same.

Other less common cancers associated with cigarette smoking are cancers of the mouth, throat and larynx, oesophagus, pancreas and bladder.

CAN SMOKING BE CONTROLLED BY PRIMARY CARE TEAMS?

Virtually all doctors and most nurses now seem to accept that smoking is dangerous. What most of them apparently do not accept is that they can do much about it. Even when they say that smoking control is an important part of care, examination of random samples of medical records (charts) shows that only a minority actually do what they say or think they do.[4] About 20% of GPs still smoke, and these are less willing and probably much less effective in giving advice to patients; it has been estimated that each doctor who smokes is worth £50,000 a year to the tobacco companies! Until recently nurses as an occupational group were heavy smokers and correspondingly ineffective health educators. This now seems to be changing, and studies of health visitors show low smoking rates.

Simply telling patients individually to stop smoking during a GP consultation results in 5% more non-smokers on follow-up one year later than in control patients not so advised. That works out at 25 ex-smokers in the first year of such a policy for each GP. A controlled study of effectiveness of structured GP counselling for smokers in Australia reported in 1986[5] has now shown beyond doubt the effectiveness of primary care counselling, if we take this work seriously. At follow-up 3 years later, 35 of 100 smokers offered counselling had become and remained non-smokers, compared with 8 out of 100 controls not offered counselling. This programme entailed a total of 6 consultations over 6 months, with discussion of personal risk profiles and measurement of the effects of smoking on lung function.

Taking smoking seriously as a disease that needs time, thought, skill, and often compassion for its defeat, is a difficult strategy to implement. We have little to go on other than personal experience, few successful models exist, and the useful literature on the subject is small. We are absolute beginners.

SMOKING, SOCIAL CLASS, AND EDUCATION

Confidence that smoking can be eliminated as a mass health risk has one sure foundation; the best-informed groups in the population are already stopping. In 1960, roughly two-thirds of all men smoked, with little difference between social classes. Between 1960 and 1975, a large social divergence appeared, particularly for men. The proportion of smokers in social class I (professional and managerial, 2% of the male population) dropped from over 50% in 1960 to about 25% in 1976 and 20% in 1982 (the last year available). Unskilled manual workers (social class V), on the other hand, dropped from over 60% of smokers in 1960 to 58% in 1976, and 49% in 1982. Women have followed the same pattern as men, except that social class V women have shown hardly any change, dropping only from 45% in 1960 to 42% in 1972 and 41% in 1982.

The most obvious reason for these differences is that people with more education are better informed. This is supported by the trend for doctors. Surveys of public opinion have shown strong social class gradients for information on all health matters. Though nearly everyone now seems to know of a connection between smoking and lung cancer, there is much less knowledge of its connection with coronary disease. In a Health Education Council Survey in 1981 about public opinion on the main causes of heart attacks, stress was cited by 53% of those questioned, though this is probably the least well established of all proposed causes, and the most difficult to treat. Smoking and obesity were each cited by 36%, lack of exercise by 20%, high blood cholesterol by 6%, and high blood pressure by 5%. Popular knowledge of risk factors in Britain is far inferior to that in the USA, although the general level of literacy is not lower here.

This difference probably reflects the fact that leading medical opinion in Britain began seriously to concern itself with coronary prevention at least 15 years later than in America.

A less obvious but perhaps equally important cause of the growing social difference in smoking may be the feelings of helplessness, fatalism, and generally low expectation in social groups who are used in times of prosperity but discarded in adversity. One of us (JTH) works in South Wales, with a general unemployment rate of 15–20%; in the Upper Afan Valley, male unemployment in 1983 was 48%, and getting worse. Changing attitudes to smoking involve changing attitudes to life. Working people, used or unused, are the most valuable asset any nation has, but they inherit deeply rooted traditions of escape through alcohol and tobacco, as well as radical assertion of their own dignity and worth. It may be that by tapping that tradition of collectivist radicalism we could solve health problems where they are in most urgent need of solution, rather than patiently waiting for knowledge to trickle down from higher to lower classes, as health educators have tended to do.

WOMEN AND SMOKING

Although risk of coronary heart attacks in young and middle-aged women has been much less than in men, much of this advantage seems to have depended on the fact that, until the Second World War, few of them smoked.

When women aged 30–44 smoke over 30 cigarettes a day, their risks of coronary heart attack are 10–15 times greater than non-smokers, about the same relative risk as in men. Recruitment of women to smoking has proceeded at about the same pace as men, but with a lag of about 30 years. If recruitment of women to smoking were to continue in the same way as it did in men, we could expect a peak in female smoking-related deaths around the year 2000. This could be averted if recruitment of women to smoking were reduced, and if more of those who smoke now were to become ex-smokers.

Though some headway has been made in reducing smoking

among women, they have fared less well than men in all except the professional class, and there has been no significant reduction in smoking among the wives of unskilled manual workers. Studies of smoking in schoolchildren show that the number of girls who smoke regularly is now approaching the number of boy smokers; at ages 15–18, 37% of girls compared with 42% of boys. In many other industrially developed countries, girls in this age-group now smoke more than boys; for example, Switzerland (46% of girls, 36% of boys), New Zealand (43%, 29%), Denmark (42%, 34%), Canada (41%, 35%), Sweden (33%, 21%), Netherlands (30%, 27%), Norway (28%, 22%), and the USA (19%, 16%).

Women not only suffer all the consequences of smoking seen in men, but also have special risks linked with oral contraception and pregnancy. Women who smoke 20 or more cigarettes a day are more than twice as likely as non-smokers to lose their child at or near birth. After birth, smoking parents (but more the mother than the father) affect their children's lungs, making them more likely to get bronchitis or pneumonia.

HEART DISEASE, HIGH BLOOD PRESSURE, AND THE PILL

Oral contraceptives have a complex relation with smoking and heart risks. They cause a small but significant rise in systolic and diastolic pressure in nearly all women (whether they smoke or not). In a few women they cause serious hypertension which can occasionally become irreversible. Both these effects may promote atheroma and narrowing of the coronary arteries and thus increase risks of coronary heart attack, and the rise in pressure makes stroke from subarachnoid haemorrhage more likely. Combined with cigarette smoking, there seems to be a synergistic effect. Pill-takers smoking 35 cigarettes or more each day have a 20-times greater risk of coronary heart attack than non-smokers. This effect may persist after stopping the pill, if oral contraception has been maintained for 5 years or more. The consequences of continued smoking should be made clear to every woman who starts on the pill, usually at an age when cigarette addiction is more a matter of social conformity than true nicotine dependence.

A COMMUNITY DIMENSION FOR THE PRIMARY CARE TEAM

To prevent stroke and coronary heart disease, customs must change. Nearly all medical and nursing training assumes that all our work is with individual sick people. This assumption is reinforced by the demands of our daily work. Every day we seem to face more patients than we can give sufficient time to, of whom most seem unmoved by personal advice; though 5% are not smoking one year after being advised to stop, 95% still smoke. Why and how should we tackle groups or even whole communities when it is so difficult to manage even our traditional task of personal consultation, and the results of this most direct of all approaches are apparently so poor?

Recruitment to smoking is imitative and conformist, depending on a powerful international image of sophistication, maturity, and adventure, projected and sustained by the tobacco companies at an annual propaganda cost of over £100 million. Second only to their own families, people turn to us, nurses and doctors, in the community in their times of trouble. We need to look afresh at our neighbourhoods to find opportunities for more locally informed, more friendly, more sensitive ways of helping people to see the truth and act on it. National organisations like the Royal Colleges of Physicians, General Practitioners and Nursing; Action for Smoking and Health (ASH), the Health Education Council, broadcasting authorities and some sections of the press, are essential but not sufficient to change custom; primary care teams are at the right level to unite theory with practice.

For example, about £60 million a year is spent by children on cigarettes, only about 12% of which comes from vending machines; the rest being sold illegally by shopkeepers. Dr N.C.A. Bradley, an Exeter GP, visited 37 local shops listed in Yellow Pages as tobacconists, newsagents, and confectioners, and interviewed them about the problem. All but 5 admitted selling cigarettes to children, one shopkeeper adding that in his opinion 'There ought to be a law about it'. Of course, there is a law; Section 7 of the Children and Young Persons Act of 1933. Enforcement depends on changing local as well as general states of public opinion so that it becomes accepted that life and health is at stake, and there is a real moral issue involved. Primary care teams are aware of the consequences of smoking in terms of personal tragedy rather than statistical abstraction, and are well placed to take local initiative to get the law known, respected, and enforced. The patients registered with a practice include a complete cross-section of local society; local government officers, borough and county councillors, teachers, clergy, active members and officers of the many organisations to be found in every well-established community. All the contacts are there to get effective decisions to extend smoke-free zones in local public areas, to get organisations to accept speakers on the smoking problem either from ASH or local primary care teams, and to ensure that councillors and members of parliament are well informed and aware that there are now more potential votes available against smoking than in favour of it. For those who want a more adventurous campaign, the Australian groups Billboard Utilising Graffitists Against Unhealthy Promotions (BUGA UP) and Movement Opposed to Promotion of Unhealthy Productions (MOP UP) offer some imaginative ideas which deserve emulation in Britain.[6]

CONCLUSION

Cigarette smoking is the most important single reversible cause of coronary heart disease, and of many other causes of premature death. Its control and eventual abolition in the local community deserves the highest priority of all preventive work by the primary care team. Big changes are needed in the way that GPs, health visitors, and community and practice nurses work, before rhetoric on this subject is replaced by action. In the absence of serious government commitment, progress depends on local initiative. Primary care teams should accept a leading role in this, as well as a responsibility to extend the traditional personal consultation to include education on the effects of smoking and ways of stopping it.

REFERENCES

1 Royal College of Physicians of London. *Smoking or health*. London: Pitman Medical, 1977.
2 Report of a WHO Expert Committee. *Smoking and its effect on health. Technical Report Series 568*. Geneva: World Health Organisation, 1975.
3 Doll R, Hill AB. *British Medical Journal* 1964; **1,** 1460.
4 Fleming DM, Lawrence MSTA. An evaluation of recorded information about preventive measures in 38 practices. *Journal of the Royal College of General Practitioners* 1981; **31:**615.
5 Richmond RL, Austin A, Webster IW. Three-year evaluation of a programme by general practitioners to help patients to stop smoking. *British Medical Journal* 1986;**292:**803.
6 Chapman S. A David and Goliath story: tobacco-advertising and self-regulation in Australia. *British Medical Journal* 1980;**281:**1187.

Chapter 5
HIGH BLOOD PRESSURE

'Blood pressure' refers always to arterial pressure, which is:

heart output × resistance of the arterial tree

Certainly less than 5%, probably less than 1% of all cases of high blood pressure are secondary to a known cause such as coarctation of the aorta or renal artery stenosis, and these will not be considered in this book. The other 95% of high blood pressure is still usually described as of unknown cause; 'essential', or primary hypertension. This is no longer accurate because, though we don't know all the causes of primary hypertension, we probably do know most of them; inheritance is certainly very important, so are obesity, alcohol, fat and potassium and probably sodium in food, depression, and probably 'stress' in at least some people.

Though raised heart output may be a feature of high blood pressure in its early stages, in established high blood pressure there is a generalised narrowing of the smaller arteries by tightening of their spiral muscle fibres, leading to raised peripheral resistance. Most antihypertensive drugs act by interfering with this mechanism.

HIGH BLOOD PRESSURE IS NOT A DISEASE: HYPERTENSIVES ARE NOT SICK PEOPLE

Figure 5/1 shows that all risks rise continuously throughout the

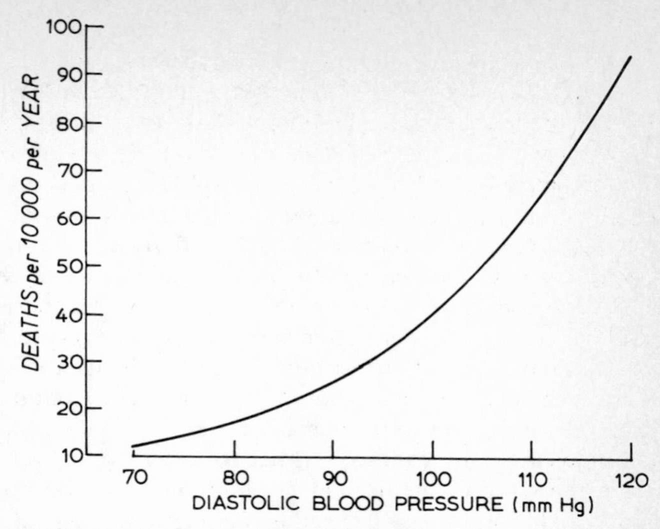

Fig. 5/1 Risk function for mortality against diastolic pressure in men 35–44 (*data from the Framingham Heart Study, Mass.*)

range of diastolic pressure, without any threshold we might use to separate 'high blood pressure' from 'normal blood pressure'.[1]

Uncomplicated high blood pressure rarely causes symptoms, but it is often associated with them. People with headaches often consult their GP, they often have their blood pressure measured, and therefore many hypertensives have headaches when they are first diagnosed. However, studies of whole populations show that headaches occur no more often in people with high blood pressure than in the general population, unless they have very high pressures indeed, around 240/130mmHg. Even then, most hypertensives don't get headaches. We have seen three patients in general practice, all found on routine testing, with blood pressures >330/170mmHg, without any symptoms whatever. In general, the true symptoms of high blood pressure are symptoms of organ damage. By that time, high blood pressure is truly a disease, and hypertensives are in the process of becoming sick people, but very few of those found by screening or case-finding in a local population will be in this group.

Why does this matter? If GPs, nurses, and others in the primary care team think high blood pressure is an illness and hypertensives are sick people, they may also believe that diagnosis and treatment of high blood pressure can depend on patients' initiative for both initial ascertainment and subsequent follow-up. If patients believe that high blood pressure is an illness, and that antihypertensive drugs are a remedy for it, they will expect to feel ill when their blood pressure is high and well when it is low, and to feel better with antihypertensive drugs than without them. Not surprisingly, they are likely to lapse their medication as soon as they feel better. They naturally assume that if they feel well, their disease has been cured, and neither medication nor follow-up is necessary.

Before the stage of organ damage, high blood pressure is a reversible risk factor, not a disease. People with high blood pressure are healthy people who need treatment (though not always with antihypertensive drugs) to stay healthy. Many, probably most, will feel at least a bit less well with antihypertensive drugs than without them. All will feel to some extent limited by their dependence on medical supervision.

HYPERTENSION AND HIGH BLOOD PRESSURE

High blood pressure and hypertension mean exactly the same thing and we therefore recommend that primary care teams stick to the traditional term 'high blood pressure', which is simpler and less ambiguous. It also leads naturally to the next question: 'How high is high?'

WHAT IS THE DIVISION BETWEEN 'HIGH' AND 'NORMAL' BLOOD PRESSURE?

Figure 5/1 shows that there is no natural division between normal and high blood pressure; for all large groups of people, the higher the pressure, the greater the risk. At pressures around 230/130mmHg, high blood pressure may become self-accelerating by destruction of the small arteries in the kidney, which, if not controlled, almost always leads to death from brain haemorrhage or kidney failure within two years (malignant hypertension). Even at these very dangerous levels, there is a wide variability between individuals. Some people can tolerate very high pressures and survive many years without symptoms, organ damage, or accelerating into the malignant phase. The trouble is, we can't predict who they will be, except to say that in general women tolerate high blood pressure better than men.

EXPERIMENTAL EVIDENCE FOR A MANDATORY THRESHOLD FOR TREATMENT

Because even severe high blood pressure rarely causes symptoms before organ damage occurs, and because the aim of treatment is to prevent organ damage whenever possible, it is now universally agreed that some hypertensives must be offered treatment on grounds of pressure alone.

This threshold for mandatory treatment can only be established by the results of randomised controlled trials, showing that total as well as cardiovascular and cerebrovascular death rates and non-fatal event rates are significantly reduced in actively treated people, compared with placebo-treated controls. We must also take into account the potential side-effects of treatment and the disadvantages of medical dependency, so that we can openly and honestly explain to patients the decision they have to make on whether to accept treatment and follow-up, which must usually continue for the rest of their lives.

For severe hypertension, in the diastolic range 115mmHg and over, several trials (most notably the first US Veterans' Administration trial) have clearly established sufficient benefit to make the treatment of all these people a matter of urgency. Practices without screening programmes will continue to miss these cases, which though relatively infrequent, are certainly not rare. The second US Veterans' Administration trial[2] seemed convincingly to lower the threshold to 105mmHg, but it was conducted on a hospital-referred population rather than one screened from the general population, and there have always been misgivings (on this side of the Atlantic, at least) about how far its conclusions could be applied to screened GP populations. All these trials showed big reductions in stroke, heart failure, and ruptured aorta, but none of them showed any convincing reduction in coronary heart deaths.

The Australian and MRC trials

For milder hypertension, the best evidence is from the Australian National Blood Pressure Study (ANBPS),[3] and the much larger and more recent British Medical Research Council (MRC) trial,[4] based on screening of half a million healthy people aged 35–64. It is unlikely that trials of this size will ever be repeated, and this is the best evidence we are ever likely to get.

Benefit in the ANBPS and MRC trials was mainly from reduction of stroke and heart failure, hardly at all from reduction in heart attacks. A huge price was paid for this benefit, not only in cash terms but in medical and nursing effort, and in entanglement of patients in all the penalties of long-term medication. The MRC trial showed that in the diastolic range 90–109mmHg, it took 850 patient-years of treatment to prevent one stroke, and there was no overall reduction in heart attacks or deaths from all causes compared with untreated controls. Such advantages of treatment as there were, were almost confined to non-smokers; benefit for those who continued to smoke was very small, a point we shall return to later in this chapter.

The HDFP and the limitations of the MRC trial

In flat contradiction to these trials was the very large US Hypertension Detection and Follow-up Program (HDFP),[5] which showed big reductions in coronary mortality, as much as 25% in some subgroups, and a 14% reduction in non-cardiovascular mortality. There were no untreated controls, and outside the USA the results of this trial were not universally accepted even before the MRC trial results were available. The design of the MRC trial is far more powerful, and in general we think its conclusions are more convincing than the HDFP.

It is possible, however, that the HDFP conclusions may apply better to those British populations which resemble the HDFP population in social composition and circumstances. Both trials were certainly socially selective, the MRC trial by mainly recruiting participants from group practices in non-industrial areas with relatively low workload, the HDFP by mainly recruiting from disadvantaged city populations, with over-representation of the black and poor. The unexpectedly large benefits in the HDFP were concentrated in these disadvantaged people. It would be consistent with the results of the Veterans' and other smaller studies if benefit were to be greatest in the people with highest risks, which the black and the poor certainly are. This important and controversial issue has been discussed.[6,7]

Another limitation of the MRC trial is its surprisingly high drop-out rate. Over the 5 years of the study, about 44% of the men and 38% of the women stopped their treatment, either by lapsing or because their doctors withdrew them. Even for the placebo-treated controls, only about a third of the withdrawals were because blood pressure rose consistently above 200/110mmHg. A drop-out rate of over 40% in 5 years is not perhaps surprising compared with other published work from hospitals, often showing annual drop-out rates well above this figure, but we have little doubt that when planned hypertension control becomes a normally accepted part of general practice, much lower drop-out rates will be achieved and results (in less heart failure and stroke) will improve.

COSTS AND BENEFITS OF UNIVERSAL MEDICATION FOR ALL GRADES OF HYPERTENSION

If (as in the USA) we define high blood pressure as all diastolic pressures at and over 90mmHg, about 20% of the adult population is hypertensive. A GP with an average list (all ages) of 2200 who decided to find and treat all high blood pressure thus defined in the age-range 20–69 (1364 people) would have a caseload of 273 patients. If we assume that each of these has to be seen once every three months, they would add 1092 consultations to the present expected total of about 6600 consultations a year for all causes.

Of people with high blood pressure, 85% lie within the MRC diastolic range 90–109mmHg, and 15% in the range at and over 110, which gives our average-list GP 232 MRC range and 41 more severe hypertensives to treat. Let us assume that treatment of more severe hypertension prevents three times as many strokes as treatment of hypertension in the MRC range (a reasonable assumption in the light of other trials), and that this zealous GP treats all of them as assiduously as they would have been treated in the trials, with the same drop-out rate. Then the positive consequence of this huge (and currently impossible) effort would be to prevent one stroke for every 2½ years of work.

A REASONABLE THRESHOLD FOR MANDATORY TREATMENT

As yet, the authors of the MRC trial have left us to draw our own conclusions, and neither they nor the editorial in the *British Medical Journal*,[8] have suggested a new threshold for mandatory treatment. In Glyncorrwg we are returning to the medication threshold of 175/105mmHg which we used until 1980 (after the Australian trial we reduced our diastolic threshold to 100mmHg), and this is what we recommend in the absence of other positive indications for treatment, mainly diabetes or evidence of organ damage.

This or any other threshold should be based on the average of at least three readings on separate days. To categorise any patient and start treatment on the evidence of a single reading is a clinical crime.

SHOULD HIGH BLOOD PRESSURE BE TREATED IN THE ELDERLY?

Treatment for high blood pressure begun in middle age should be continued in the elderly, though often lower doses are needed, and treatment should certainly be reviewed and not enforced blindly. As more middle-aged hypertensives are detected and treated, the number of old people presenting for the first time with high blood pressure will fall.

Until recently there was little evidence for or against starting treatment for the first time in the elderly. We now have convincing evidence from the European Multicentre Working Party trial[9] and from John Coope's multicentre trial in general practice[10] that treatment begun in the elderly is effective in preventing stroke and heart failure, though once again it is ineffective in preventing coronary heart attacks, and there is no reduction in all-cause mortality.

CAN HIGH BLOOD PRESSURE BE PREVENTED?

The belief that high blood pressure can be prevented rests on the fact that populations exist in which high blood pressure is unknown, and blood pressure does not rise with age. All these populations live in relatively isolated communities with very low salt intake, and all of them are thin. When these people move to cities, get fatter, and eat more salt and more meat, their blood pressures rise, and rise with age, just like people who have always lived in urbanised and industrially developed countries.

Obesity

There is convincing evidence that young men who are overweight are more likely to develop high blood pressure as they get older, and young men with high blood pressure are more likely to become overweight. No one has yet conducted the critical (and extremely difficult) experiment to see whether weight reduction in youth can prevent later high blood pressure, but action of this kind can certainly do no harm and may be effective. Blood pressure does fall in middle-aged men and women who lose weight, but the effect is small.

Salt and diet

There have been several carefully conducted, random controlled studies on the effects on blood pressure of substantial but not extreme reductions in salt intake. These have shown a small effect (a reduction of 5–7mmHg diastolic pressure) in people with blood pressures high enough to need antihypertensive drugs, but no significant effect in people with borderline hypertension in the range 150/90–169/99mmHg.[11] It's possible that salt restriction of this degree (to less than half the sodium intake usual in Britain) would be effective if it were maintained for months or years rather than a few weeks, or perhaps throughout childhood. One of us (JTH) has been involved in three studies of sodium restriction, and his impression was that restriction to below 5g sodium (about 85mmol) daily was difficult for nearly all patients, and for the research team who conducted the study and tried it out on themselves. Other researchers have claimed otherwise, saying they find low sodium diets readily acceptable to their patients. We suggest that readers put themselves on a low sodium diet, verifying their intake by sending at least three 24-hour urine collections for measurement of sodium output. They can then decide the matter for themselves. Without verification by measurement of 24-hour sodium output, subjective impressions of reduced salt intake mean nothing at all.

Other changes in diet look more promising. Vegetarian diet, excluding meat, fish and poultry, but including milk products and eggs, causes a significant fall in blood pressure in normotensives. Stringent reduction in dietary fat (to 23% of energy intake, compared with the usual 35% or so) causes a greater fall, higher in both hypertensive and normotensive people. Vegetarian diets contain less fat, so these effects are likely to be related. The case for a national diet with less meat and a higher content of cereals, fruit, vegetables and fish is now strong, and more convincing than the case for big reductions in dietary salt.

Relaxation and reduction of stress

Not surprisingly, patients who learn to relax also lower their blood pressure, but there are two big questions about this as a method of treatment. Can relaxation for say 30 minutes a day cause a permanent lowering of blood pressure? And, if so, is such treatment feasible in practice?

There is some persuasive evidence that borderline hypertensives can lower their blood pressures by relaxation techniques, though it is difficult to prove this in controlled trials. Those who believe that high blood pressure is usually or always induced by 'stress' are naturally attracted to the idea, because they think they are dealing with the cause rather than merely treating an effect, but the evidence on this is not wholly convincing. This book is not the place to discuss current theories on the cause or causes of essential hypertension, but the stress theory is probably less popular now among medical scientists than it was 10 years ago.

Though teaching relaxation techniques is time-consuming, it is suitable for group work and patients can quickly learn to treat themselves. There seems to be no doubt that if primary care teams are interested enough to learn these techniques, their application in practice would be feasible, probably effective for mild hypertension, and not necessarily any more time-consuming than supervision of drug treatment.[12] None of us has any experience of them, so they are not dealt with further in this book. (A full account of Chandra Patel's technique is given in *Hypertension*, 2nd edition 1987.)[7]

Two warnings need to be borne in mind by those who do use these techniques. First, most borderline hypertensives are found to have lower blood pressures on follow-up for the first 6–9 months at least, even if they are not treated at all. In the Australian trial nearly 2000 placebo-treated controls had diastolic pressures 95–109mmHg (sustained through two readings) at entry, but 47% of them had diastolic pressures less than 95mmHg at follow-up 3 years later, without any active treatment. So the first warning is to remain suitably sceptical about the apparent effects of any treatment for mild hypertension for at least 5 years.

The second warning is just the opposite. In the same trial, 12% of the placebo-treated controls showed a rise in diastolic pressure up to or beyond 110mmHg at follow-up after 3 years. Mild hypertension may not remain so, and a rise in pressure accelerating to dangerous levels can occur unpredictably in anyone in this group. Hypertension at or over a diastolic threshold of 110mmHg has never been convincingly controlled by moderate sodium restriction, weight reduction or relaxation, without medication in any controlled trial; on present evidence blood pressure at this level always needs treatment with anti-hypertensive drugs.

CONCLUSION

Control of high blood pressure is the most popular starting point for control of coronary disease, but there is no convincing evidence that it is effective for this purpose. It is certainly effective for control of heart failure, stroke, and in preventing a further rise in blood pressure to more dangerous levels; these are the main justifications for blood pressure control in middle age. If high blood pressure could be prevented in youth by changes in diet and by controlling obesity, this might have a bigger effect on coronary heart mortality than treatment of high blood pressure in middle age, but there is still no conclusive evidence of this.

The organisational tasks of blood pressure control are a good introduction to the more complex tasks of preventing coronary heart disease and stroke by controlling other risk factors, starting from familiar procedures more readily acceptable to present primary care teams; but control of smoking, blood fats, and obesity are likely in the end to prove more effective targets.

Effective treatment and follow-up of high blood pressure depends on understanding by the whole primary care team, and by patients, that uncomplicated high blood pressure is not a disease, and that hypertensives are not sick people. Decisions about treatment should be explained to and shared with patients. Unpleasant and harmful side-effects must be taken into account in deciding whether to begin or to continue treatment with antihypertensive drugs, as well as the relative risks of leaving high blood pressure untreated.

Control of other risk factors in hypertensives, particularly smoking, is often more important than control of high blood pressure itself.

REFERENCES

1 Kannel WB, Gordon T. *The Framingham study: an epidemiological investigation of cardiovascular disease*, section 26. Washington DC: Government Printing Office, 1970.

2 Veterans' Administration Co-operative Study Group. Effects of treatment on morbidity in hypertension II: results in patients with diastolic blood pressure averaging 90 through 114mmHg. *Journal of the American Medical Association* 1970;**213**:1143.

3 Australian National Blood Pressure Management Committee. The Australian therapeutic trial in mild hypertension. *Lancet* 1980;**1**:1261.
4 Medical Research Council Working Party. MRC trial of treatment of mild hypertension: principal results. *British Medical Journal* 1985;**291**:97.
5 Hypertension Detection and Follow-up Program Co-operative Group. Five-year findings of the HDFP. *Journal of the American Medical Association* 1979;**242**:2562.
6 Hart JT. Role of the family practitioner. Clinical aspects of essential hypertension. In *Handbook of hypertension*, vol.1, p. 463 (ed. Robertson JIS). New York: Elsevier, 1983.
7 Hart JT. *Hypertension*, 2nd edition. Edinburgh: Churchill Livingstone, 1987.
8 Breckenridge A. Treating mild hypertension. *British Medical Journal* 1985;**291**:89.
9 Amery A, Brixho P, Clement D et al. Mortality and morbidity results from the European Working Party on high blood pressure in the elderly trial. *Lancet* 1985;**1**:1349.
10 Coope J, Warrender TS. Multicentre trial of treatment of hypertension in the elderly in primary care. *British Medical Journal* 1986;**293**:1145.
11 Grobee DE, Hofman A. Does sodium restriction lower blood pressure? *British Medical Journal* 1986;**293**:27.
12 Patel C, Marmot MG, Terry DJ et al. Trial of relaxation in reducing coronary risk: four year follow-up. *British Medical Journal* 1985;**290**:1103.

Chapter 6
OBESITY AND DIABETES

Obesity, maturity-onset diabetes, high blood cholesterol and physical inactivity are all connected with each other, as well as being well-established risk factors for coronary disease in their own right. Obesity and diabetes are also important risk factors for stroke. Each of these factors is more likely in the presence of the others, so they are not independent, and correction of one may sometimes be more usefully approached through correction of another. For example, the first step in reducing high blood cholesterol should be to reduce body-weight. These relationships are complex and often difficult to understand, but the interconnection that underlies this complexity can be used to devise relatively simple, unified solutions.

OBESITY: DEFINITIONS AND MEASUREMENT

Much of the information in this chapter is drawn from Garrow's book *Treat obesity seriously: a clinical manual*[1] which we recommend to all primary care teams.

Obesity is not easily defined in a practical way. The simplest and least inaccurate way to range a population of various heights and weights into a single distribution is to use Body Mass Index (BMI), also called Obesity Index, Ponderal Index, and Quetelet's Index (see p. 158):

$$\text{BMI} = \frac{\text{kg}}{\text{m}^2}$$

Weight is measured in kilograms, and height in metres.

Why use such an unfamiliar formula at all? You have only to look at patients to see whether they are fat, and that's the trouble; in planned work, which depends on initial screening of records followed by screening of selected patients, you can't look at the patient, all you have is the record. Nine times out of ten this will contain some weights, but few if any heights, so there is no way of ranking for obesity and defining your treatment categories. Routine recording of heights in all patients is a relatively simple procedure, since for practical purposes height does not change after age 20, and therefore needs only to be recorded once.

Figure 6/1 can be used to make a rough estimate of BMI without the bother of calculation.

Figure 6/2 shows the relation of BMI to death rates from all causes, a U-curve in which excessive thinness also has a mortality.[2]

At roughly BMI 30, death rates for those who are too fat begin to exceed death rates for those who are too thin. This is therefore a practical dividing line between 'cosmetic' and 'medical' obesity, though of course the cosmetically obese may be on their way to medical obesity, particularly if their parents are fat. The definition of medical obesity used from now on in this book is BMI=30+.

'Desirable weight' lies in the range BMI 20–25, because this range is associated with the lowest death rates from all causes. The interval BMI 25–30 we call 'cosmetic' obesity.

Giant obesity

What we call 'giant' obesity, and Garrow calls Category III, starts arbitrarily at BMI 40. These people are very fat indeed, at least 45kg (roughly 100lb) above maximum desirable weight.

Giant obesity is a serious, intractable, and often tragic problem. The results of all forms of treatment are usually disappointing, though that is not a good reason for not trying. Almost certainly the most effective treatment is to give early and sustained support to people at BMI 30–39, so that they never cross the line into giant obesity. Management of giant obesity is

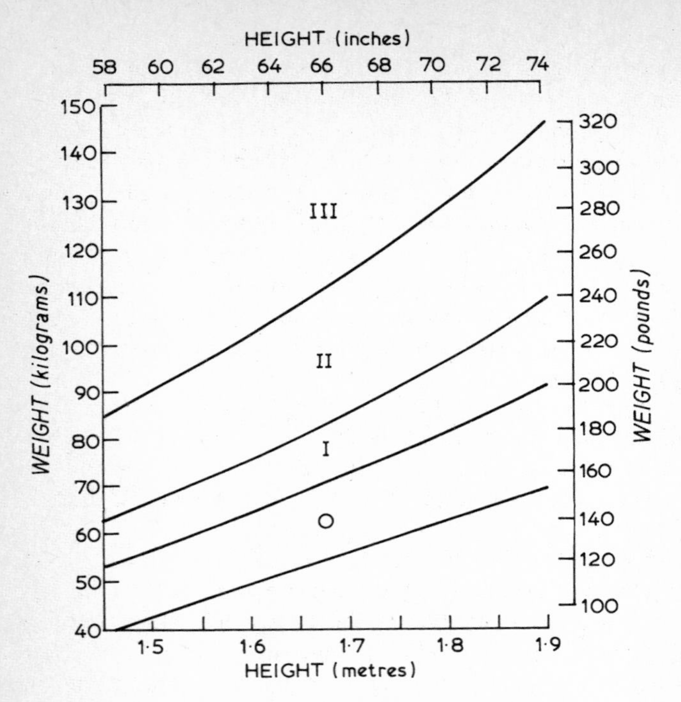

Fig. 6/1 Relation of weight defining the desirable range (0), and grades I, II, III obesity, marked by the boundaries W/H^2 = 25–29.9, 30–40, and over 40 respectively (*after Garrow*[1])

outside the scope of this book, and readers are referred to Garrow's excellent section on the subject.

WHY DOES OBESITY MATTER?

Death rates from all causes are much higher for fat people, and risks are less in those who control their weight. Obesity has a bigger effect on death rates in the young than the old; for people 10kg (about 23lb) or more overweight, death rates are 46% higher than average at ages 15–34, 30% at 35–49, and 18% at 50–65. Very fat people who survive over 65 have an almost

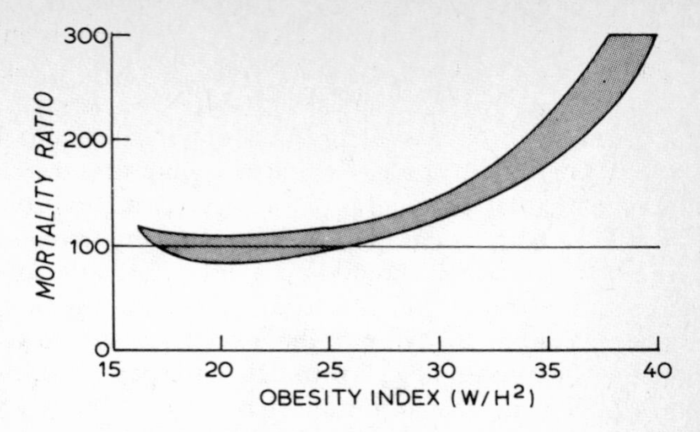

Fig. 6/2 Relation of obesity index W/H^2 to mortality ratio. Average mortality = 100 (*data of Seltzer, 1966*)

average life-expectancy (though they may be very disabled), their obesity is particularly resistant to treatment, and so, as with other risk factors, it's sensible to concentrate effort on the young and middle-aged.

What do they die of?

Fat people are at higher risk from all forms of surgery. They are more likely to get gallstones, hernias, and injuries that require surgery, are more difficult to diagnose quickly and accurately with such conditions as strangulated hernia or gut perforation, are more likely to go into heart or respiratory failure, and are much more likely to develop diabetes with all its circulatory complications. With or without diabetes, they get more coronary disease (particularly angina) and strokes. Long before they die, they tend to be seriously disabled by degenerative arthritis of the hip and knee, leg oedema and leg ulcers, impaired lung function, and difficulty in taking even the slightest exercise.

Epidemiologists have long argued whether obesity is in itself a cause of coronary heart disease. Since obesity is linked with other risk factors for coronary disease, such as high blood pressure, high blood cholesterol, diabetes, and physical inactivity, if all these are taken into account and abstracted from the equation, the solo part for obesity is small or even negligible. But this is statistical trickery; obesity almost never appears solo, and its relationship to risk factors is causal. Action to control obesity reduces blood pressure, controls glucose intolerance, reduces blood cholesterol and promotes exercise. Obesity is an easier target to understand than the use of antihypertensive or antidiabetic drugs, which should logically be used after obesity has been tackled rather than before, particularly in the mild hypertensives and maturity-onset diabetics generally picked up by screening or case-finding. For practical purposes, control of obesity is the second most important step in prevention of coronary heart disease, after control of cigarette smoking.

DIABETES

Diabetes is five times commoner in obese men than in men of average weight, and nearly eight times commoner in obese women. Control of obesity is very effective; two-thirds of all non-insulin-dependent (maturity-onset, or type II) diabetics can recover a completely normal glucose tolerance test after 6 months of good dietary control, without the use of antidiabetic drugs. People with a history of diabetes in parents or siblings are at particularly high risk, but onset of diabetes in them can be prevented by anticipatory weight control.

Fat people need more insulin than thin people, and their pancreases have to work harder to produce it. It seems that people with a family history of diabetes tend to have a pancreas that is easily exhausted by chronic overproduction of insulin, and the most physiological way to conserve their pancreatic function is to reduce body weight. The cause of diabetes in these people is obesity, so treatment should first of all be directed at this cause, with resort to oral antidiabetic drugs only if a reduced-energy diet fails to control blood glucose levels.

Dietary control should not be considered as failed if it has never been seriously tried. Patients will diet successfully only if they understand the nature of diabetes, the composition of foods, and a few simple facts about the conversion of other foods into blood glucose, as well as the procedures for measuring blood and urine glucose. This learning process was found at one London teaching hospital to require an average of 4 hours, individually or in small groups. In most hospitals, and in nearly all general practices, nothing like this amount of teaching is offered, so it is not surprising that dietary treatment is so commonly thought to have failed. It is much easier to prescribe pills.

DIABETES AND HIGH BLOOD CHOLESTEROL

In countries with generally high blood cholesterol, diabetic men have a 2 or 3 times higher coronary risk than non-diabetics, and diabetic women have a 5 or 6 times higher risk. Stroke risk is also increased, by about 25% in women and a bit less in men. Few diabetics now die from uncontrolled diabetes itself: overwhelmingly, they die of its complications, chiefly coronary disease, stroke, damage to the aorta and leg arteries, and circulatory damage to the kidney leading to renal failure. For every one of these, the other risk factors for arterial disease are shared; smoking, high blood pressure, and high blood cholesterol.

The coronary risk of diabetes is probably not a direct effect of high blood glucose, but of the high blood cholesterol levels usually associated with it in people eating 'Western' diets. The medically-prescribed diabetic diet traditional up to the late 1970s, high in animal fats and low in cereals and potatoes, tended to push up blood cholesterol still further, increasing atheroma and coronary risk. Modern diabetic diets, with fats reduced below 30% of total energy intake and increased fibre (wholemeal cereals, vegetables and fruit) are effective both in reducing blood cholesterol and in controlling non-insulin-dependent diabetes.

The diabetics in any practice are the group most vulnerable to arterial disease, who can benefit most from early diagnosis and assiduous long-term care, and suffer most if these are neglected.

REFERENCES

1 Garrow JS. *Treat obesity seriously: a clinical manual.* Edinburgh: Churchill Livingstone, 1981.

2 Seltzer CC. Some re-evaluations of the build and blood pressure study 1959 as related to Ponderal Index, somatotype and mortality. *New England Journal of Medicine* 1966;**274**:254.

Chapter 7
BLOOD CHOLESTEROL AND EXERCISE

HIGH BLOOD CHOLESTEROL

We have already seen that most people in Britain have a high blood cholesterol compared with countries like Japan, with a low average blood cholesterol and a very low incidence of coronary heart disease. It is sometimes said that many people get coronary heart attacks who have none of the three major risk factors, but in fact this is rarely true; with few exceptions, their blood cholesterols are normal only in that they are within two standard deviations of the average for Great Britain.

Cholesterol measurements made in hospital laboratories are usually reported as within or above a 'normal range', defined between the bottom 5% and the top 5% of all values found in the local or national population. My (JTH) local laboratory, for example, gives the normal range for total cholesterol as 3.8–6.7mmol (147–260mg)/dl at ages <40, and 3.8–7.8mmol (147–300mg)/dl at 40 and over. At a consensus conference in the USA,[1] moderate risk was defined from a threshold of 6.2mmol (240mg)/dl, and high risk from a threshold of 6.7mmol (259mg)/dl, well within the 'normal' limits set by my local laboratory. If the word 'normal' is to have any real meaning, how can we apply it to levels of blood cholesterol clearly associated with disease?

If we are concerned with high blood cholesterol values not because they are unusual, but because they cause disease, we should accept that the appropriate normal reference populations are not in Britain, with an average blood cholesterol of 6.2mmol (239mg)/dl, but around the Mediterranean and in the Far East, with average blood cholesterols between 4.1mmol (160mg) and 5.2mmol (200mg)/dl.

BLOOD CHOLESTEROL AND DIET

The real question is how to shift the entire population distribution of blood cholesterol down towards the Japanese or Mediterranean pattern, which we know to be associated with low risks of coronary heart disease. The most effective way to achieve this would probably be to reduce the average total fat intake to about 30% of all energy intake as recommended by the Health Education Council, together with an increase by 50% in the proportion of fat derived from vegetables and fish.

PRECISE DIAGNOSIS OF HYPERLIPIDAEMIAS

Specialised hospital clinics attempt precise diagnosis and treatment of the various ways in which blood fats may be raised, the many Fredericksen types and subtypes. We suspect the complexity of this classification has caused more bewilderment than enlightenment among GPs, and has tended to restrict the task of hyperlipidaemia control to a handful of specialists who cannot possibly help more than a few people.

Fat circulates in blood on its way from the gut to the liver, and from the liver to other parts of the body where it may be used to lay down energy stores, or deposited in the artery walls as atheroma. Such fat as is needed for immediate energy is metabolised to glucose in the liver. Fat circulates in blood as triglyceride, cholesterols, and free fatty acids (FFAs). All of these may contribute to coronary atheroma, and FFAs may also play a fatal part in the events following infarction of heart muscle. Cholesterol circulates in different forms, separable with an ultracentrifuge into high (HDL) and low (LDL) density fractions. Different proportions of these fractions have been thought to have different risk implications; HDL seems to have a protective effect, reflecting mobilisation and transport of cholesterol, whereas LDL increases risk, reflecting deposition of cholesterol as atheromatous plaques on the arterial lining.

These complexities should not be allowed to confuse the simple advice needed by the vast majority of people with high blood cholesterol. Total blood cholesterol can now be estimated quickly, cheaply, and accurately using clotted blood from non-fasting subjects on an auto-analyser, whereas the manual methods used up to the early 1970s were often inaccurate. Indeed, recent developments suggest that dry auto-analysers, using a single drop of capillary blood, could be in routine use in the GP's surgery within the next 5 years, giving accurate cholesterol values at the time of consultation. The capital cost is already around £3,500 and the unit cost for each test about 50p.

HEREDITARY HYPERCHOLESTEROLAEMIAS

Roughly 1 person in 500 carries a single gene for familial hypercholesterolaemia, resulting in a blood cholesterol of at least 8mmol(310mg)/dl and a correspondingly high relative risk of coronary disease. People carrying 2 such genes, who are extremely rare, nearly all die from coronary disease under 30 years of age, mostly in childhood, unless their high levels of blood cholesterol can be brought down by very strict dieting and generally unpleasant drugs. All of these children could be identified if the first degree relatives of all cases of coronary disease under 45 were screened for blood cholesterol. Control of familial hypercholesterolaemia in children is a heartbreaking business; even in skilled hands, results are generally poor. Inherited disorders of this kind account for less than 1% of all cases of severe hypercholesterolaemia.

LOW-CHOLESTEROL OR CHOLESTEROL-LOWERING DIETS?

An illusion shared by most of the public, many nurses and some doctors is that cholesterol in food is the main source and determinant of cholesterol in blood. This is not so. Cholesterol is a main chemical pathway for the construction, transport, and destruction of a variety of cell structures throughout the body, and its level in blood bears no simple relation to its concentration in food. Dietary fats and oils of all kinds, as well as carbohydrates and some proteins, contribute to the level of blood cholesterol. There is a lot of evidence that some fats are more important than others in promoting high blood cholesterol and atheroma. Unsaturated fats, with numerous free hydrogen bonds, cause less atheroma than saturated fats. Unsaturates are derived generally from plants and fish, saturates are derived from farm animals, either in meat, or in milk and its products. High fish consumption, typical of Japanese diet, reduced coronary death rates by 50% in one Dutch trial,[2] and other studies have shown a dramatic reduction in blood LDL cholesterol and triglycerides after addition of fish oils to diet.[3] This may be the most important new development in control of coronary disease during the next few years.

HIGH RESIDUE, HIGH FIBRE DIETS

Vegetable foods contain varying amounts of woody or gummy materials which are not absorbed through the gut, but may modify the way in which other nutrient foods are handled. These very different substances are loosely grouped together as 'fibre'. Some commonly available high fibre (or 'high residue') foods are raw fruits and vegetables, cooked beans and other pulses, and wholemeal bread. Very generally, these foods increase transit time for food in the stomach, reduce transit time in the rest of the gut, and improve blood glucose control in diabetics, probably by evening out the absorption of nutrients over time. There is some evidence that they may reduce total blood cholesterol, and other more convincing evidence that they may substantially reduce the risk of coronary heart disease, not necessarily by this mechanism. They also help to prevent diverticulitis and gallstones, and may help to prevent appendicitis.

Most high-residue foods take a lot of chewing, may be rather boring to eat, and increase the volume though not usually the pungency of 'wind'. People who can resist the temptation to eat other more appetising foods with more concentrated energy (mainly fats, sugars, and meats) may therefore tire of eating more quickly and eat less, and thus attain the first objective of all cholesterol-lowering diets, a negative energy balance with weight loss. Effective high-fibre diets depend mainly on increased intake of wholemeal bread, cooked beans, peas and other pulses. Other vegetables lose most of their 'fibre' when cooked, but large raw salads are effective. High-bran foods such as breakfast cereals and diet biscuits are often made more palatable by added sugar, which defeats the whole object of the exercise. Did you know that 'All Bran' contains 15% of sugar by weight, and muesli 26%?

The Health Education Council now suggests a target of 30g fibre daily for adults, a 50% increase on the present average diet containing 20g. For comparison, vegetarians average about 42g daily. This figure could probably be attained fairly easily, mainly by increased consumption of wholemeal bread and pulses.

SUGAR

Sugar provides concentrated energy in an attractive and palatable form, often combined with fat (as in cakes and chocolate). Reduction in sugar intake is almost the only point that all the many fashionable reducing diets have had in common, and rightly so. Elimination of added sugar is one of the quickest and easiest ways to reduce energy intake, without much disturbance of normal meals. Sugar in tea or coffee is an obvious target. Less obvious and often overlooked are soft drinks, pops, and so-called 'health drinks' such as Lucozade.

ALCOHOL

Like sugar, alcohol is a concentrated source of energy, and is often ignored as a fat-promoter. It now accounts for 5–7% of the energy intake in an average adult diet. Reduction in beer intake is an important part of any plan for weight reduction in most men.

There is now good evidence from many sources that small

quantities of alcohol (up to 2 glasses of wine, 1 pint of beer, or 1 double measure of spirits) have a favourable effect on the proportions of high and low density cholesterol fractions, and probably reduce coronary risk. The results of surveys in different parts of the world are remarkably consistent in finding a J-shaped curve for coronary death rates, with a slightly higher rate in total abstainers than in moderate drinkers. Heavier drinkers (more than 4 drinks a day) have a substantially higher coronary risk, probably because of raised blood pressure. There is now no doubt at all that high alcohol intake is a common and important cause of high blood pressure, and that periods of extra heavy drinking often precede a stroke.

A COMPLICATED STORY WITH A SIMPLE ENDING

Despite the complexities of the evidence on diet and coronary disease, practical conclusions can be fairly simple. People under 50, particularly if they have a bad family history or are known to have a total blood cholesterol >7mmol(270mg)/dl, should take the following four steps:

1. Reduce energy intake with the aim of attaining desirable weight for height (BMI = 25).
2. Reduce fats of all kinds by one quarter.
3. As far as possible, replace dairy and meat fats by fats and oils derived from vegetables and fish.
4. Increase vegetables and fruits, particularly those eaten raw, eat wholemeal bread, and increase the proportion of bread in the diet.

Over 55 there is no convincing evidence that reductions in blood cholesterol reduce risk.

CHOLESTEROL-LOWERING DRUGS

Drugs are of limited value in reducing blood cholesterol.

Cholestyramine (Questran) is a bulky (24g daily) nauseating anion-exchange resin which binds cholesterol in the gut and blocks its metabolism. It causes a lot of gas both ends and is generally poorly tolerated, but it can reduce blood cholesterol by about 28% in patients who take all their medication and also adhere strictly to a cholesterol-lowering diet. It is very expensive.

Clofibrate (Atromid S) has been much more widely prescribed and is much easier to use. Taken over several years it doubles the incidence of gallstones, without any overall reduction in deaths. Its use seems to be justified only in people with Fredricksen type III hyperlipidaemia, and even then, only as an adjunct to diet.

Neither of these drugs is a substitute for diet, and none should be considered until dieting is well established and its effect on blood cholesterol has been measured.

HIGH BLOOD CHOLESTEROL CAN AND SHOULD BE TACKLED

The US Lipids Research Clinics trial (already referred to, p. 67) has shown conclusively that reduction of high blood cholesterol does prevent a significant number of coronary deaths. Its subjects were men in the top 5% of the distribution of blood cholesterol in USA (the top 5% in Britain would have even higher cholesterols), average age 48, average blood cholesterol 7.5mmol(292mg)/dl. Men treated with diet plus cholestyramine had a fall of 14% in blood cholesterol, compared with 5% in the controls on diet alone. The coronary death rate over seven years was 19% lower in the test group than in the controls. Side-effects of cholestyramine were generally unpleasant, and were complained of by 68% of men after one year, and 25% after seven years.

The results of this trial are a powerful argument, not for routine use of cholestyramine (even in this top 5% of the cholesterol distribution) but for planned reduction in blood cholesterol for all men under 55 with blood cholesterols at this sort of level, by dietary means. The evidence already quoted of a downwards shift in average US blood cholesterol levels of about 12% suggests that sustained dietary advice to the whole population, using all available channels of information and persuasion including doctors and nurses, is just as effective as medical advice to subgroups at exceptional risk.

Since the first step in all cholesterol-lowering programmes is weight reduction, and since effective reduced-energy diets also tend to have a cholesterol-lowering effect, primary care teams should first of all concentrate on the visible, cheaply and easily measured, and readily understood problem of obesity under 55, mounting a broad campaign for healthier eating by the whole population.

EXERCISE AND CORONARY DISEASE

That dietary fat isn't everything is supported by the fact that among wealthy people, consumption of animal fats has fallen rather than risen throughout this century, although coronary heart deaths only began to occur commonly about half-way between the wars. This can be partly explained by recruitment to cigarette smoking, but another likely explanation is the decline in physical exercise, both at work and in leisure time, accompanying mechanisation of production and transport.

This protective effect of regular exercise could be exerted in several ways, not mutually exclusive. Regular vigorous exercise may reduce blood pressure, may improve the efficiency of the heart so that if infarction occurs it is less likely to be fatal, may improve glucose tolerance, may reduce total blood cholesterol, and raise its high and reduce its low density fractions. None of these effects is large, nor have they always been convincingly confirmed by subsequent studies. Exercise may also act indirectly by encouraging a more general change in lifestyle towards better diet, no smoking, and less alcohol. The most convincing evidence of a protective effect of exercise suggests that sustained high-level energy expenditure has its own important effect on coronary risk, which is independent of other major known risk factors and is not mediated through them.

ENERGY BALANCE AND ENERGY THROUGHPUT

An abiding truth that has survived all the swings of slimming fashion is the cruel fact that unless energy expenditure exceeds energy input, body weight will not fall, though given regular exercise there may be a useful replacement of fat by muscle.

Physical exercise is not the only way the body uses energy. Simply to maintain the human machine in a state of idleness requires about 100 calories (0.4MJ) an hour. If instead of lying down doing nothing you get up and jog for an hour, your energy consumption rises to 300 calories (1.2MJ); not a lot out of a daily consumption of 2500 calories or so. Miners working at a non-mechanised coalface in 1952 were found to use an average of 3660 calories a day (15MJ) compared with an average of 2800 calories a day (12MJ) for colliery clerks, a difference of only 860 calories between very hard labour through a whole working day, and the sort of office work generally prevalent today.

It is therefore not surprising that increased energy expenditure through exercise is generally much less effective as a slimming tactic, than a lower-energy diet. Nor is there any convincing evidence that exercise reduces appetite or raises resting energy expenditure (basal metabolic rate (BMR)). The necessary point of departure for everyone who wants to be leaner (which includes nearly everyone with a high blood cholesterol) is to accept that though fat people may be convinced they eat no more than thin ones, and are sometimes right, the only way they will lose weight is to eat less energy than they need, for long enough to attain a lower weight, and then permanently stabilise their energy intake at this lower level.

That being said, exercise is still the most important aid we have to weight control by dieting. This help comes less from shifting the balance of energy intake and output, than from the cultural effect of regular exercise. The reasons we eat as we do, that we like some foods and not others, that being bloated with one food we may turn eagerly to another, seem to be extremely complex, and based as much on acquired habit as on simple gut reflexes.

Eating differently is a big change in behaviour, and regular exercise, particularly in a group, assists that change by effects on mood, confidence, self-regard, and an increased will to live fully. Certainly our experience has been that groups using regular exercise as well as diet are more successful in losing weight and maintaining their loss, and have fewer drop-outs, than groups that concentrate on diet only.

Common sense as well as some experimental data suggest that energy throughput may be important to health as well as energy balance. 'Use your health', said George Bernard Shaw, 'even to the point of wearing it out. That is what it is for.' Unlike fine wines, health doesn't improve with storage.

REFERENCES

1 Consensus conference: lowering blood cholesterol to prevent heart disease. *Journal of the American Medical Association* 1985;**253**:2080.

2 Kromhout D et al. The inverse relation between fish consumption and 20-year mortality from coronary heart disease. *New England Journal of Medicine* 1985;**312**:1205.

3 Phillipson BE et al. Reduction of plasma lipids, lipoproteins, and apoproteins by dietary fish oils in patients with hypertriglyceridemia. *New England Journal of Medicine* 1985;**312**:1210.

Chapter 8
SECONDARY PREVENTION

Secondary prevention is management of survivors of heart attacks and strokes so as to reduce the risk of a second and worse event.

Obviously these survivors are at extremely high risk, and this has both advantages and disadvantages. The return for effort invested is relatively good, in that the difference in outcome between well-managed and neglected patients is high, much higher than for people who have not yet suffered obvious arterial injury. It is nearly always worth trying. The impact on the overall health and longevity of the whole practice population is small, but good work on this high-risk group does a lot to give the team credibility in its potentially more productive work of primary prevention, as well as to raise morale within the team itself.

Secondary prevention is much more a part of traditional medical care than preventive work directed at people without symptoms, and is a good potential starting point for improved practice performance by setting objectives and auditing their attainment. Despite its apparently traditional nature, it is still poorly performed in most demand-led general practice, because patients demand so much less than they might usefully receive.

SECONDARY PREVENTION OF STROKE; CONTROL OF HIGH BLOOD RESSURE

Figure 8/1 compares the effect of good and bad management of hypertension in people who have already had one stroke;[1] it speaks for itself.

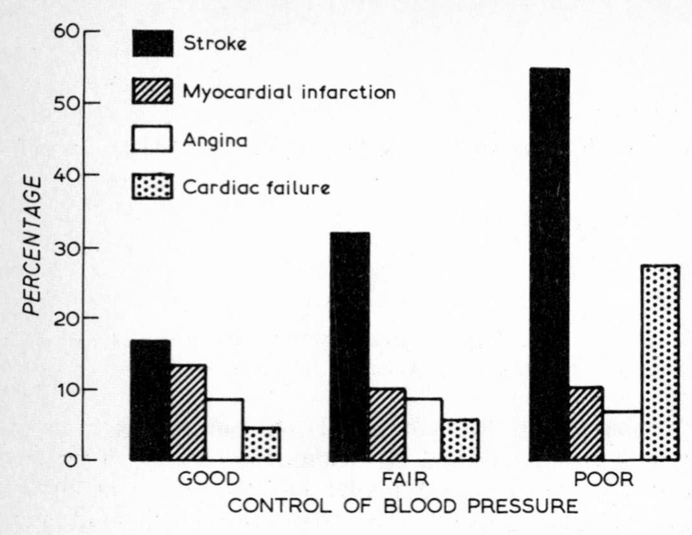

Fig. 8/1 Frequency of cardiovascular and cerebrovascular disease in relation to control of blood pressure

Good control of hypertension is mandatory in anyone who has had a stroke with a raised blood pressure, even from a threshold of 150/90mmHg, unless brain damage has been so severe that useful recovery is impossible. Unexpected useful recoveries do occur even from very severe strokes, though prolonged unconsciousness makes this very unlikely. In our experience most victims of major stroke have had previous evidence of vascular brain damage, often minor and apparently transient. Patients and carers need to be alert for these, and to respond by stricter control of blood pressure and more assiduous monitoring.

Raised blood viscosity

Other risk factors for stroke need evaluation in each individual case. Smoking does increase risk, but to a far smaller extent than in coronary disease. Raised blood viscosity, with a *packed cell volume* (PCV, haematocrit) of 0.5 or more, is an important additional risk, and very common in industrial working-class communities with a lot of chronic lung damage. There have been no controlled trials of the effect of reducing PCV by venesection, though this is a simple and safe procedure well worth considering in the individual case. More important is to remember that diuretics will reduce plasma volume and thereby raise PCV, and so should be avoided wherever possible for people whose PCV is already high. Small doses of aspirin (one adult-sized tablet a day) have a marked effect on platelet adhesiveness and probably have a worth-while effect in reducing risk of further stroke from emboli detached from atheromatous carotid arteries, but there have been no conclusive results from controlled trials.

Alcohol

Another major and hitherto neglected risk factor for stroke is alcohol. High alcohol intake is the commonest explanation for a *mean corpuscular volume* (MCV) >95fl, usually a better indicator in the stroke age-group than *gamma glutamyl transferase* (GGT), but the best indicator is simply to take a detailed history of normal weekly alcohol intake. Though, like smokers, drinkers tend systematically to underestimate and understate their intake, their answers generally give a better indication of the extent of the problem than any more objective indicators like MCV and GGT. A stroke is a horrifying event to both patient and relatives, and providing the causal relationship between alcohol and stroke is explained, compliance is usually good.

SECONDARY PREVENTIONOF HEART ATTACKS[2]

Smoking

By far the most important step to take during and after a heart attack is to stop the patient from smoking. It is essential to take action during the acute phase of the illness, when patient and relatives are most receptive to advice. One Swedish study[3] showed that 77% of patients surviving a first attack were smokers. Over half of these (57%) stopped smoking before discharge from hospital, and fewer than 10% of these resumed smoking during two years of follow-up; but of the 43% who did not stop while in hospital, less than 10% gave up during the following two years. The death rate in those who did not stop was twice as high as in those who did. These figures were almost exactly replicated by a similar study in Dublin.[4]

The moral is to get in quick, before the patient returns to 'Marlboro Country'. A visit by a member of the primary care team before the patient leaves hospital can be very effective. Hospital medical staff have plenty else to do, and often omit to give specific, sustained, and personalised advice on smoking.

Beta-blockers

There is now no doubt at all that some beta-blocking drugs given during the year following a myocardial infarct reduce mortality in survivors by 25% during that year, probably by protecting the heart against lethal disorders of heart rhythm.[5] Because this effect does not apparently continue after the first year, the long-term protective effect is small, but this 25% reduction in the first year is well worth having, and beta-blockade should be considered in every survivor in whom there is no contra-indication, mainly heart failure or reversible airways obstruction. Baseline measurement of *peak expiratory flow rate* (PEFR) is essential to reveal latent asthma which is surprisingly common. The effect is proven only for propranolol and timolol, and may be confined to these.

Aspirin

There has been a lot of conflicting evidence about the preventive effect on coronary disease of drugs affecting platelet adhesiveness. Evidence in favour of dipyridamole (Persantin) is unconvincing, but evidence for the protective effect and safety of small doses of aspirin (1 adult tablet of soluble aspirin a day) is good, and has been accepted by the cautious US Food and Drugs Administration.

Anticoagulants

Secondary prevention of myocardial infarction in the elderly by assiduously controlled anticoagulant treatment, with warfarin for example, reduced 2-year mortality by 44% in the very impressive double-blind randomised trial in the Netherlands,[6] to which British doctors (both GPs and specialists) seem strangely resistant. It is difficult to understand why this is still not being generally done, where there are no obvious contra-indications (mainly, a past history of gastro-duodenal ulcer or gut bleeding). Treatment should be maintained as long as good anticoagulant control is feasible.

REFERENCES

1 Beevers DG, Fairman MJ, Hamilton M et al. Antihypertensive treatment and the course of established cerebrovascular disease. *Lancet* 1973;**1**:1407.
2 Evans AE. Secondary prevention after myocardial infarction. *Lancet* 1986;**2**:150.
3 Wilhelmsson C, Vedin S, Elmfeldt D et al. Smoking, hypertension, and physical activity after myocardial infarction. In *Acute and long-term medical management of myocardial ischaemia* (eds Hjalmarson A, Wilhelmsen L), p. 265. Molndal, Sweden: Haessle.
4 Mulcahy R, Hickey N, Graham I et al. Factors influencing long-term prognosis in male patients surviving a first coronary attack. *British Heart Journal* 1975;**37**:158.
5 Breckenridge A. Should every survivor of a heart attack be given a beta-blocker? *British Medical Journal* 1982;**285**:37.
6 Sixty-plus Reinfarction Study Research Group. Risks of long-term oral anticoagulant therapy in elderly patients after myocardial infarction: second report. *Lancet* 1982;**1**:64.

PART THREE: HOW TO DO IT

Chapter 9
TALKING AND LISTENING TO PATIENTS

Effective patient education depends on ability to know your pupils well enough to give them appropriate and understandable information. The information you wish to give may concern medication, lifestyle or the next appointment: whatever it is, they must be able to understand, remember and act on that information, if it is to bring about any change in health.

'HOW DO YOU FEEL?'

How do patients feel when they come to the doctor?

Many studies have sought to discover the answer to this question and have described patients' feelings of nervousness, frustration and being hurried during consultations. If we consider the patient's progress through the health centre or surgery, step by step, we can perhaps understand better not only where these feelings come from, but what we might do to relieve them.

RECEIVING PATIENTS

This is what the receptionist does. She has a responsibility both to doctors and other staff for the smooth day-by-day running of the organisation, and also to patients, for answering their questions, ensuring that they are seen by the person they want, and that they have the necessary information for the next step they need to take.

This is a difficult, 'pig-in-the-middle' job, and receptionists have acquired the unkind title 'dragon at the gate'; that may be what patients expect to meet when they approach the receptionist's window.

To be fair to receptionists, their job is a difficult one, not only because they have to mediate between doctor and patient, but also because they usually have to do many things at the same time. A receptionist was observed in one practice sending a patient through to the doctor while answering the telephone, looking for a prescription to give to another patient and handing a second doctor some notes. It is hardly surprising that patience with patients wears thin!

Patients cannot be expected to understand all this, and what they see and hear may make them feel they will have to fight for a fair hearing. This apprehension and possibly aggression can be carried over to their interactions with the doctor. Whether or not that happens, an unsatisfactory encounter with the receptionist will disturb and upset patients, long before they meet a doctor or nurse.

The art of reception has always been underestimated in health care. Large hotels and big businesses take reception seriously, insisting upon adequate training in communication as well as office organisation. At last general practice is catching on: courses and videos for receptionists are becoming available which highlight the importance of effective communication with patients.

Even with adequate training, receptionists can only be as good as doctors allow them to be. If they have instructions never to bother doctors, to protect them from home visits and extra patients and instantly to meet the doctors' every need (rather than the patients') then it will be just about impossible for the patient to beat the dragon.

Having enough receptionists on duty will help everyone, and might be worth the financial investment in greater job satisfaction for receptionists, smoother running of the practice and, most importantly, fewer disgruntled patients.

The design of the reception area can also influence the quality of communication between receptionists and patients. If receptionists have to peer through a tiny window to speak, it is difficult to establish eye contact, or even to hear what is said. Perhaps any window at all is a barrier stating that 'we (the health care team) have to be protected from them (the patients)'; but unfortunately sometimes that's true; we are not angels, and nor are the patients.

Waiting

Waiting rooms are a give-away. Look at any waiting room, and you can judge how keen the provider of the room is to keep your custom.

Think now of the waiting room in your surgery – is it designed to relax patients, make them feel welcome, warm and comfortable while they wait? Your waiting room is the first indication to your patients of the concern which you have for them; patients usually spend longer in the waiting room than anywhere else, and the quality of their waiting affects their tempers and anxiety levels as well as their willingness to return for more waiting when asked to.

Imagination, together with care for those who wait, can be as effective as cash investment in turning your waiting room into an inviting place. Look carefully at some waiting rooms which you like, and use some of their ideas. You may not be able to swap your upright chairs for sumptuous armchairs, but perhaps they could be grouped around a small table instead of in rows. Is your waiting room warm enough? Do you have a selection of recent reading material? What about a patients' lending library, so that books on health topics they have got well into while waiting can be taken home and finished? What about a play area for children? Is that a feasible project? You will be surprised at how many patients will respond to an appeal for second-hand toys, playpens, children's books, or small chairs.

THE CONSULTATION

If you have been for an interview for a job, you will probably have been nervous. The longer you had to wait for the interview, the more nervous you felt. When you entered the inverview room you were perhaps faced by a panel of people behind a table, or by a powerful boss seated at an imposing desk. Maybe your nervousness made you think less clearly, and the answers you gave to questions were not nearly as good as the ones you thought of later when your mind was calm and clear.

On the other hand, you may have interviewed somebody else for a job. When you're the interviewer it's difficult to imagine how nervous the interviewee may be. The room, the desk, the people and the subject under discussion are so familiar to you – your common daily round – that it becomes almost inconceivable that any of them could be frightening.

When you work in general practice as a nurse or doctor you find that patients frequently present the same, or similar, symptoms – for example, a headache, a cough, backache, fatigue. Because rare diseases are rarely encountered it is likely that many of these symptoms will indicate a self-limiting ailment, which probably doesn't need medical attention anyhow. Much of general practice is made up of this sort of work, often referred to by professionals as 'trivia'. It's familiar work to both nurses and doctors and so not frightening, just as the surgery or treatment room is familiar, the papers on the desk, the equipment in the cupboards. To patients each encounter with the doctor or nurse puts them in the position of an apprehensive interviewee. Nervous patients may not be able to express themselves well, may forget to ask something they want to know or may not be able to concentrate well enough to remember what they are told.

To communicate effectively with your patients you have to understand and appreciate their feelings, put them at their ease and then ensure that you use the consultation time effectively, enabling your patients to express themselves, ask questions, learn, and remember what they have learned. Without it, any hopes of compliance with diets, smoking cessation, exercise programmes or return visits are in vain.

'Come in and sit down'

The way you greet patients conveys your interest (or lack of it), just as your greetings to friends and relatives do. The same skills are needed to convey warmth, welcome and interest to both friends and patients, even though the level of interest may be different. Compare the following examples:

CONSULTATION A

Doctor: (*writing notes of previous patient and without looking up*) Come in and sit down.

Patient: Good morning, Doctor.
(*few moments' silence*)

Doctor: Ah – yes – it's Mrs Jones, isn't it?
(*Picks up notes from pile.*)

Patient: Well, actually I'm Mrs Smith, Doctor.
(*nervous laugh*)

Doctor: Sorry, yes, must be in the wrong order. Well, what's the matter today? (*Looks briefly at patient then starts looking through her notes as she speaks.*)

CONSULTATION B

Doctor: (*Rising from desk, indicates chair, smiles and looks at patient.*)
Hello, Mrs Smith. How's the family?

Patient: Fine thanks, Doctor.
(*Smiles, looks at doctor, sits.*)

Doctor: (*Sits and maintains eye contact with patient.*)
How can I help you today?

It's easy to see not only from the words used but from the way in which the doctors behaved towards their patients that the warmth and interest expressed were vastly different. In example A the doctor did not know who the patient was, made no attempt to put her at her ease and appeared to be more interested in her notes than in her.

The B doctor clearly has better social skills – remembering something about the patient (her name and that she has a family), showing interest in her by making eye contact and showing warmth by rising to greet her and smiling.

Can you improve your welcome? Make a checklist of things

that seem important in example B, and see how your own greetings compare. You will probably be surprised to find that your greeting technique varies very little from one patient to another.

Taking a history

In a consultation concerned with changing lifestyles your main aim must be to discover the individuality of your patients. You want them to tell you all about their lives; their habits, illnesses, family, stresses, employment, attitudes and aspirations. Although some people, given half a chance, will talk about themselves at length, many find it difficult.

Firing structured questions at patients may produce the answers you're seeking but is less likely to reveal the underlying attitudes which influence compliance with suggested changes in lifestyle. The question 'Do you smoke, and how much?' reveals some useful information, but 'Have you ever tried to give up?' as a follow-up opens the door for all kinds of anecdotes, some of which will be helpful to the listener in planning possible cessation strategies with the patient. For example: 'Well I did give up once for two weeks, but then I lost my job and the wife gave me a cigarette 'cos I was upset.' This response contains a wealth of information for the health teacher: the patient was able to give up smoking, he may still be unemployed, his wife smokes, and they both smoke in response to being upset.

Open-ended questions, that is questions which don't simply invite yes or no answers, are useful as a method of getting people to talk about themselves. In order to glean the information you need, either about an illness or about a lifestyle, you have to listen actively to what your patient is saying, remembering what is said and prompting when necessary.

Open-ended questions, because they require active listening to be of any use, and because they invite patients to talk about themselves, have patients as the centre of attention during the consultation. You may think this is always and obviously the case, but that is not so. Consultations often have the doctor or nurse as the main focus, because they do most of the talking and make the plans and the decisions. Sometimes the illness presented, or a procedure, are the centre of attention, patients are people being overshadowed by the clinical interest they offer.

Making an effort to think of each part of a consultation (the welcome, then Subjective information, Objective information, Assessment, and Plan: SOAP) as patient centred makes patients feel at ease, wanted and understood and makes communication easier for both of you. It also improves the chances that your patients will comply with treatment, because if you accept patients as equal partners in their own health care, then both of you will be better able to accept that there are two levels of outcome for consultations: what you advise, and what your patients do with that advice.

MAKING PLANS

Accepting your patients as partners in their health care means accepting them as equals. Their talents differ from yours, their social, educational and economic backgrounds may be worlds away from your own, but they are experts on their own lifestyles and can tell you more about their physical, mental and emotional feelings than anybody else. Their human experience is as valid as yours: to succeed as a health educator you need to value your patients' stories and appreciate their importance for both of you.

If, one weekend, you planned to go for a picnic and thought you'd like to go with a friend, it would be foolish simply to turn up at her house to collect her on the appointed day without first finding out whether she wanted and was able to go with you. Making plans in which others besides yourself are to participate, requires that the views, availability and willingness of other prospective participants are first canvassed.

That seems so obvious that it scarcely seems possible that it needs saying, and yet health professionals are often guilty of making unilateral plans:

> 'Right then, Mr Jones, come back tomorrow to have that dressing changed.'
> 'Here's a diet sheet, Mrs Smith. I think you should lose some weight.'

'I'm going to alter your tablets – stop taking the blue ones and start these new pink ones, four times a day after meals.'

It is often difficult to strike a balance between knowing best what your patients should do and asking them what they are willing and able to do. Not allowing your patients to have any say in the decisions you feel qualified to make about their health means that no matter how sound your advice, they may not heed it.

Just as our plans which involve friends' participation will fail if we do not include them in the planning, so our attempts to prescribe for our patients will fail if they are left out at the planning stage. Taking into account the patient's commitments, mealtimes, hours of work, family life, leisure pursuits, helps us to appreciate the cost of changes which we ask our patients to make; not, perhaps, financial expenditure, but cost in terms of choice, choosing one way of life instead of another.

If we suggest that a patient needs a chest *x*-ray, does that mean he must lose time (and money) from work? If your patient is a heavy smoker and you want him to give up, will it affect his relationship with his mates at work? Or his wife at home? We are not suggesting that you should never give advice or information to your patients, but that you should also ask for their opinion about the advice and whether it is feasible; and, having asked for their opinion, listen to it and include it in plans made together.

Doctor: I'd like you to take these capsules 4 times a day before meals. There you are (handing prescription). Come back when the capsules are finished.

This is one possible way of making a plan but compare it with this:

Doctor: I'd like you to take these capsules 4 times a day before meals. Can you manage that?
Patient: Well – mmm – the thing is, I don't have 4 meals a day.
Doctor: No, of course, that's a silly way for me to put it! What I

mean is that you should take the capsules at least half an hour before you eat anything or an hour after you've eaten anything. They don't work if you take them with milk either, or with some stomach medicines. Can you manage to take them half an hour before breakfast, lunch and supper and again when you go to bed?

Patient: I can manage breakfast and supper and bedtime, but it might be difficult to take the lunchtime dose because I'm at work then. Could I take 2 at bedtime instead?

Doctor: Good idea. Why don't you give that a try and come and see me again in a month to tell me if they're helping clear your skin?

In the second conversation, the doctor is offering greater explanation and encouraging the patient to express his views. To some extent the doctor is self-critical too, which demonstrates that he feels he is on a par with the patient, ready to revise his own plan in the light of new and useful information.

Basing your plans on what both of you agree the patient may manage will result in greater satisfaction all round; you will get the desired change in behaviour, and your patient will be further motivated by a sense of achievement.

FURTHER READING

Byrne PS, Long BEL. *Doctors talking to patients: a study of the verbal behaviour of general practitioners consulting in their surgeries*. London: HMSO, 1976.

Chapter 10
MANAGING PREVENTION

In this chapter we suggest ways of using records to store information about your patients' risk factors and of setting about finding and helping those patients most at risk of early heart disease or stroke.

THE USES OF RECORD SYSTEMS

Preventive work depends on planned care of the whole population registered with a practice, sorting it into various groups by age, sex, and the measured risk factors required for effective anticipatory care. As we are planning to avoid future events like strokes and coronary disease, we can't use those events to identify the patients who need care, as we have done in the past. Nor can we approach the whole population indiscriminately. We have to have some way of ranking priorities, initially sorting out patients without actually having to see them. The way to do this is to use the records to represent the patients, so that the first stage of screening for risk data is to screen the records, not the patients.

This requires that the records accurately represent the patients, that they contain all the data relevant to anticipatory care, and that this information is readily accessible.

The change from records that merely assist the GP during consultation, to records that give an accurate risk profile to the whole team in the patient's absence, is hard work but worth while. This change involves the non-medical practice staff in setting it up, and opens the record to use by the nurses and other staff who will be recording most of the risk data from now on.

Things you'd like to know about your patient

If the purpose of your record system is to enable you to plan anticipatory care for your patients, then you need to know, as well as SEX FAGS COPS (see p. 7), their occupations, perhaps their postcodes, telephone numbers, and other information which you would usually be able to ask directly, in demand-led care.

Where and how can you record all this information so that it will be easy to find (a) when the patient attends the surgery and (b) if you wish to send for at-risk patients for screening procedures?

ORGANISATION: LLOYD-GEORGE AND A4

Have a look at what you've already got in the way of records. You will probably think first of the familiar red or blue NHS medical envelopes issued to every general practitioner in Great Britain for each patient. These were first introduced by Lloyd-George in 1916, so we shall refer to them from now on as Lloyd-George records. These have now been in use, almost unchanged, for 70 years. They're cramped, too small to accept hospital letters unfolded, and it's difficult to structure the information in them; that is, to create an information system in which there's a known place for everything, and everything is in its place. It can be done, but only with great effort.

On the whole, we think the effort required to restructure Lloyd-George records might be better spent in converting to A4 records, essentially on the hospital pattern. These offer much more space, hospital correspondence can be filed unfolded, and the book-type design offers better possibilities for structuring information. Over half of GPs in Scotland have converted to A4, and the Scottish Home and Health

Department (SHHD) still pays for the new stationery for all GPs willing to use it.

GPs in England and Wales who want A4s have to fight for them, and only about 5% of practices have them now. In our experience, you can get them if you rightly refuse to accept no for an answer. We have not heard of any practice anywhere which, having converted to A4, has regretted doing so. On the other hand, there is almost universal agreement that A4 does create more clinical work by revealing deficiencies. We are therefore justified in asking Family Practitioner Committees (FPCs) to meet the fairly small part of the cost represented by the actual purchase of new stationery, and in health centres, to provide the necessary extra shelving or carousels.

The costs of A4 are the clerical time needed for setting them up and transferring selected data from Lloyd-George, the medical time needed to extract major events from Lloyd-George and set up an A4 summary sheet, the nurses' or dispensers' time needed to transfer treatment data, and the costs of filing these much bulkier records. They can be housed cheaply in lateral files on the wall, using wooden shelves which can be built by a local carpenter, but this takes up a lot of wall space and won't be feasible for many practices. Though many Lloyd-George records are housed in double rows in metal cabinets which will accept A4, these require a lot of extra space for pulling out. The alternative is to use rotating carousels. These are expensive, but take up less space than Lloyd-George records filed laterally or in drawers. FPCs in many areas have accepted the cost of providing these in health centres. Because A4 costs money, the final decision will rest with GPs, and even they may face opposition from partners. Like it or not, many teams will still have to make do with Lloyd-George.

Whether you keep the Lloyd-George envelopes or decide to invest in A4, some pruning will be helpful. With a guillotine or one of the much cheaper and more efficient sliding razor-blade trimmers, hospital letters can be cut down to the text, but if you do this be careful not to lose hospital reference numbers. Many hospital letters are repetitive, and a lot of other material accumulates which is obviously redundant. But, before throwing this out, bear in mind the possibility that important risk variables may be contained in some of them, particularly old laboratory reports. For example, reports of full blood counts, which are rarely of much clinical use, nevertheless contain *mean corpuscular volumes* (MCVs) which are a useful indicator of alcohol problems, a much commoner cause of high MCV than B12 deficiency. *Packed cell volume* (PCV) is a risk factor for stroke, and you may sometimes want to identify people with PCVs of, say, 0.5 or more. Total blood cholesterol is included in many auto-analyser results and will be useful for screening, and blood urea and creatinine results indicating kidney function are also likely to be important.

Normal results are just as important as abnormal results: we are looking for ways of ranking risk in which the whole distribution of values needs to be known. Practices which have shaped up their records, with or without conversion to A4, and subsequently proceeded to an efficient system of anticipatory care, frequently find that they have been hasty in throwing overboard information during the initial shaping-up process. Probably the safest procedure is to keep all the old material, but get it into date order (with the latest data on top), and save the culling for later on when you have a few years' experience of what data you actually need.

Identification data

These are the name, address, date of birth, and anything else you want on the outside of the record to help to identify, categorise, and contact your patients. For example, you may record telephone numbers, car ownership, or clinical categories indicated by coloured patches. Lloyd-George envelopes have a small space for occupation (rarely completed), and on A4 there is space for this on the inside of the folder. It is worth considering entry of postcodes with the address, not only to speed up mailing, but also because the Office of Population Censuses (OPC) can provide mortality figures based on postcodes, so that you can compare data for your own practice with figures for the general population in your area.

Summary cards and sheets

The essence of anticipatory and preventive care is to escape from the traditional episodic style of consultation, by steadily building up a documented life story about the patient's health. The first step in this is to have a concise summary of significant life events, preferably as the front page of the record.

Lloyd-George-sized summary cards are available from the Royal College of General Practitioners, with structured positions for entry of data, or you can get summary cards from the local FPC, blank on one side and with immunisation data-slots on the other. These can be used to record the main illnesses and life events, as well as a family history, on the blank back side. For A4, there is a standard blue summary sheet available with plenty of space for subsets of information such as family history.

Who will write the summaries? All the hospital correspondence and all the consultation entries have to be scanned for evidence of events of lasting significance, a process which on average will require about 10 minutes for each patient; often less, but occasionally a lot more. This is the main bottleneck in upgrading records. Some GPs claim to have solved it by giving their patients self-administered questionnaires to fill in their life histories themselves. Readers over 50 years old can try recalling their own life histories, and attempt to attach a year to each major event; we doubt if they will do this with either ease or accuracy. The job could perhaps be given to a very experienced nurse or receptionist with a good general knowledge of medical terms, working to guidelines from a GP. Others have delegated it to trainees, but in our experience, a trainee with enough confidence, balance, and knowledge of the non-hospital world to do this job accurately and safely, no longer needs training.

Generally speaking, we think this is unavoidably a job for the GP with whom the patient is registered, who should, after all, be responsible for getting an accurate past history if anyone is. This will mean long hours of overtime, probably over a year or more, but at the end of this the quality of the records and the medical care received by patients should be strikingly improved. All the GPs we know who have done this, regard it as a turning point in care of their patients.

Filing correspondence

Pick, at random, 10 sets of notes from your shelves, and look at all those letters and sundry items which make the file bulge and make re-insertion of the notes in the envelope almost impossible. Could some of them be summarised on one piece of paper? Could the hospital correspondence be filed separately, leaving more space in Lloyd-George for summary, treatment, and continuation cards? On A4, there is a separate file at the back.

Here is a suggested checklist for organising your letters:

Put letters and investigation results in date order, earliest at the bottom, latest at the top.

Consider filing them in separate groups, one for hospital correspondence and the other for investigations.

Several letters relating to the progress of one episode of illness could be summarised retrospectively, or the best hospital or referral letter could be selected.

Irrelevant material can be discarded, for example, a written request from a patient for a repeat prescription, but you should discuss within the team what your policy is going to be on this and perhaps run a short period of a week or two before you reach a final decision.

Letters and investigation results should be treasury-tagged through a punched hole rather than stapled, for ease of adding and subtracting material, and access.

What about the notes made by practitioners and receptionists? Can you read them? Is there too much or too little information about each patient?

Recording treatment

How far back do you have to look to see what drugs the patient is taking, whether they have worked, or whether they have caused unpleasant side-effects? Can you tell, only by searching the record and without asking patients, what treatment they are supposed to be having?

For A4, there is a green laboratory reports sheet which can be easily adapted to function as a treatment sheet, either for all prescriptions, or for long-term medication (repeat prescriptions) only. For Lloyd-George, a repeat prescription card is available from FPCs. Not only severe drug reactions, but any reason for not repeating a drug (that it doesn't work or that the patient cannot tolerate even its recognised and normal side-effects) should be entered in some easily accessible place.

Recording the consultation

Roughly 5% of practices now type their continuation notes, usually by the doctors using small hand-held dictaphones, which are then used by a secretary for typing on to Lloyd-George continuation cards or A4 sheets. This can be an excellent arrangement if a quick turn-around of the notes can be guaranteed. It will break down if it results in records not being available when they are needed for urgent patient care or home visits.

Anyone who has read a number of GP notes will know that their style and content are as varied as those who write them. Here are two examples encountered by one of us:

> To come for smear test next week. Problems with son – he is being chased by group of Pakistani men and boys but what he's done she doesn't know. She refuses to let him wear skinhead boots because when he does it provokes them – so he goes to school in trainers. Even had to get the teacher to take him to school as he raised so much aggro and was almost frightened to go. Much of this could be related to her symptoms. (Describes a consultation which was a follow-up of one by another GP, when investigations were started following two episodes of tunnel vision in a 32-year-old woman.)

> Rpt. 1 and 2
> Quite wheezy at present but is moving to P—— with his Alsa-

tian, Jack Russell, cockatoo and 2 canaries having sold house in W——. Staying with friends temp. then moving back to daughter if can. Refer Dental Hospital. (Male, b. 1917, chronic asthma.)

Individuality, perhaps even eccentricity, can be amusing and delightful, and who would wish to lose the occasional smile? However, some agreement is necessary on the way in which information which goes into the notes is recorded.

Many practices now use some variant of the problem-orientated record system first devised by Lawrence Weed. The chief features of this are that the patient's most important problems, or the problems most significant for planning care, are listed in date order by year on a summary sheet, and the continuation notes are structured in a definite sequence indicated by the mnemonic SOAP. This stands for.

S (subjective; what the patient tells you);
O (objective, what the practitioner observes or measures);
A (assessment; diagnosis in any dimension, not necessarily clinical, but some brief indication of the nature of the problem as you then see it);
P (plan; treatment in the broadest sense, not only drugs, but any other action required by anyone).

Use of this standard sequence makes it easier to extract information, and means that retrospective study of the records can be done relatively easily by other, often less trained, people.

The following minimum standards for records seem reasonable:

Notes should be legible.

There should not be so much information recorded that it smothers vital details, nor so little that another practitioner has no idea of the patient's problem or the outcome of the consultation.

It should be easy to identify drug therapy, and the date and quantity of the last prescription.

Any information relating to risks of future disease should be recorded in such a way that it is easy to see (e.g. underlined in red, highlighted with a felt-pen, or indicated elsewhere in the notes).

Beware of putting too much information on the record envelope, whether A4 or Lloyd-George. If records are taken on home visits, as they should be if you stick to the principle that when major decisions are taken the records should always be available, they will have a shorter life. In our experience, they rarely last more than 10 years if patients are seen fairly frequently, and often last less than 5. When the outsides have to be changed, you don't want a lot of information on them which also has to be re-entered.

The process of streamlining your notes in this way may seem tedious. There are two points which might spur you into action:

1 You might employ and train a clerk to undertake much of the tidying. You will have to think about confidentiality here, and at many other points. All practice employees should have, as part of the written contract of employment which is now a legal requirement for GPs, a clear understanding that all they see in the record is strictly confidential, and that any breach of this will result in instant dismissal. Much risk data concerns behaviour, and is in some ways more vulnerable to gossip than more traditional clinical material. Confidentiality must be apparent as well as real, and this should affect choice of employees. While it is tempting to make use of the various government schemes for occupying the time of unemployed school leavers, a perpetual rotation of these through the practice doing various clerical tasks which nobody else wants to do may pose a serious threat to confidentiality, as well as being bad employment practice. It is better to think in terms of taking suitable school leavers for initial employment on this task and subsequently employing them in an expanded practice team.

2 You will actually have begun your search for the high risk patient, because in perusing the records you will notice the patients who have defaulted from treatment, who have not been seen for a long time, whose registration is incomplete so that the practice is not being paid for them, or who have been previously noted as having one or more high risk factors.

Special ways of recording

Having organised your existing records so that they give you easy access to their contents, you are now ready to tackle the question posed at the beginning of this section; where on the personal notes are you going to record the risk information about each patient? This is an important question, because the information must be easy to enter, easy to find, and must be kept up to date.

The age and sex of your patient can be seen at a glance from the outside of the notes, while other pertinent factors have to be given space inside, and possibly outside too. Some of the information you're after needs continual up-dating, while some of it will be permanent. A lot of thought and probably some pilot experiment will be needed to decide where and how to record data so that entries need only be made once and in one place, and yet be easily retrieved. No perfect solution is possible without computer assistance, and few of us will have that during the next 5 years at least. Meanwhile, we have to compromise between what we ideally wish to have, and what we actually can have, bearing in mind the exaggerated thrift of some partners, the conservatism of some practice staff, and other ugly realities most of us prefer to forget.

One solution is a periodic health maintenance entry in the continuation cards or sheets, concise, comprehensive, and highlighted in some way; perhaps outlined in a red box, or perhaps using a specially-made rubber stamp for a checklist entry, which makes it easily recognisable.

You might decide not to make such entries on the conventional continuation sheets, but on a flowsheet of some kind, limited to recording information on preventive work, on diabetes, on hypertension, on obesity, or anything else that requires indefinite follow-up. On A4, there is a standard sheet for immunisation data with plenty of space for other periodically recorded screening data such as BP, smoking, or weight. You might record figures of systolic and diastolic pressure, or HbA1c, or weight, graphically on close-ruled graph paper, so that both care-givers and patients can easily see favourable or unfavourable trends. You can draw lines along the graph to indicate a target level for treatment. The trouble with these is that they always require either entry of data in two or even three different places, or run the risk of isolating the data from the general care of the patient, because doctors and nurses seeing the patient for other reasons rarely refer to them.

Both Lloyd-George continuation cards and A4 continuation sheets are available from the FPC in more or less unlimited quantities, and there is no reason why you should not get a local printer to overprint them in any way you want. If you do this, remember to have a pilot trial of the first draft of the form you intend to use. Those who plunge straight into a printed form without a pilot trial end up realising that they have made some disastrous error which cannot be corrected because they already have 10 000 of their first impulsive design. Figure 10/1 shows a good example.

Colour coding

To make it easy to extract all the records of a particular risk group, mark the front of the envelope in some special way.

The Royal College of General Practitioners (RCGP) has approved the following standardised colour code for some common conditions, which can be used both on the records themselves and on age/sex register cards. These have been in fairly widespread use since the late 1960s, and it's probably a good idea to stick to them as far as you can to ensure uniformity with other practices. The RCGP colour codes are:

Blue = hypertension
Brown = diabetes
Yellow = epilepsy
Black = suicidal depression and drug dependence

HEART ATTACK AND STROKE RISK CARD

Name M/F

Date		Initial Blood Pressure	
D.O.B.		Mean if applicable	
Weight		Height	

Smoker		Cigarettes		Pipe		day, since 19
Non-smoker		Never		Stopped 19		

Relevant Family History	
Own Occupation or Partner's Occupation	

Diabetes	Yes		Insulin		OHD		Diet	
	No							

Oral Contraception	Current		Past		Never		N/A

Date									
Blood Pressure									
Smoking Change									
Weight Change									
Oral Contraception Change									
Other Change									

Notes

Fig. 10/1 Heart attack and stroke risk card (*reproduced by permission from the Oxford Heart Attack and Stroke Project funded by the Chest, Heart and Stroke Association*)

In some practices the notes of all patients who smoke cigarettes are marked with a coloured patch. Patients see this applied and are rewarded by changing to a new signal when they mend their ways. The problem here is that things that are stuck on may have to be removed, and if the adhesive is any good it is likely to mutilate the record when it comes off. A solution for this is to have one colour for 'at risk', and another colour, applied on top of the first, when the risk is removed. The records of, for example, diabetic and hypertensive patients, are commonly marked in some such way on the outside of the notes, thereby alerting receptionists, and nurses and doctors.

These conditions are not always fulfilled. The coloured markers have to be placed on the outside of a record at a point where they are easily visible in whatever filing system is used. On Lloyd-George records, if the records are filed in drawers, the colour indicators must be on the top edge of the record. If they are filed laterally on shelves or in carousels, the indicators must be on the outside edge, on the side. If A4 records are used, they have to go on the spines. Coloured metal clips are useless, they always get knocked off.

The only way to do it is with coloured plastic tape, available in all the primary colours, as well as gold and silver, and red and white, black and white, and blue and white chequers. Though all these are available one way or another, any particular colour is frequently out of stock, and it is worth laying in a store of whatever you have decided to use, with generous provision for periods of famine in which one particular colour is simply not available from any source. Of course this system only works if everyone in the practice knows about the marking system, and cares about it and believes in it.

Negative indicators

These colour code systems are ideal for a practice in which the initial shaping-up of records and establishment of a data system is already accepted into routine practice. However, at the first stage, when most of the data is missing and most practice effort is going into obtaining initial data from something like two-thirds of the patients, a more appropriate method is to use a coloured cardboard or plastic insert into the Lloyd-George envelope, sticking out a couple of inches so that it is easily seen, and removed when the data has been collected. For example, if, as in most practices, less than half the population at risk has had a blood pressure recorded during the past 5 years, when you are going through the records you simply put a coloured slat into the record envelope of everyone for whom the information is missing. Then whenever a patient consults, and the receptionist, nurse or doctor sees that a coloured slat is present in the envelope, this signals that measurement of blood pressure is required. Once the information is obtained, the slat is removed. This method is particularly effective for the large majority of practices which choose to record their initial information by 'natural recruitment'; that is, recording data as and when patients consult at the practice premises for whatever reason.

Of course, the data collected need not be limited to blood pressure. Providing someone is available to obtain the information, all or nearly all major risk data can be obtained at the same time. Strips of coloured card measuring about 5cm (2in) across, and long enough to protrude from the Lloyd-George record by about 5cm (2in), can be made very cheaply by any local printer.

A slightly more expensive but more durable alternative is coloured resin-laminate (Formica), which you can get cut up into suitable strips by any do-it-yourself shop. These slats can be used over and over again for any data-collecting process on which the practice decides to embark. Obviously they can only be used for an envelope-style record, they can't be used for A4; they are the only reason we can think of for clinging to the Lloyd-George envelope.

For A4 there seems to be no other way than to put a sticker on the spine in one colour to signify 'job to be done', and then overlay this with another coloured sticker signifying 'job completed'. If you do this, as with all other stickers on the spines of A4, make sure that you put a fairly generous length of plastic strip on to the cardboard jacket. Short lengths quickly come loose and flap about, eventually dropping off the record. Here again, any ideas you have for new record design should be subjected to pilot experiment in your own practice, as unexpected snags nearly always arise which can be corrected before you go into full-scale production.

Having looked at the practical problems relating to the keeping of records let us now turn to workload involved in terms of human capacity.

WORKLOAD

Seriously to discuss changes in lifestyle and permanent major risks requires not just 10 rather than 5 minutes, but half an hour or more, probably on several occasions. This is a point in favour of having special sessions for screening during which patients can be given appointments every 20 or 30 minutes. Trying to offer this style of consultation on a case-finding basis can result in disgruntled patients and anxious doctors and nurses. If you have screening and follow-up clinics outside your normal surgery times you may find this also solves the problem of space, because you can use your usual rooms at new times.

Long sessions are not the only way. In Glyncorrwg we have shown that a lot can be done by structuring patient education over repeated short visits, acquiring and imparting a bit more information each time, though even then it must be structured, or the work agreed upon never gets done. Even so, this is continually threatened by other, more urgent calls on professional time. With enough staff (but who has enough staff?) special sessions are easier to protect from the chronic state of emergency in which GPs and practice nurses normally live.

Spreading the load

The realistic alternative is to stop thinking only in terms of either doctors or nurses, traditionally trained to work as fast as possible in anticipation of the next unforseeable emergency, and think instead about creating new job descriptions, probably but not necessarily filled by a nurse with traditional training, deliberately geared to a much slower pace, with a prolonged consultation time, perhaps 20 or 30 minutes.

Throughout this book we have suggested that nurses have undeveloped potential as providers of anticipatory care. This is partly because nurses are often more thorough than doctors in working to a protocol, and therefore likely to be better at structured screening of groups; partly because nursing as a philosophy is a broad church, perhaps encompassing counselling and teaching more naturally than medicine (though things are changing); and partly because it's possible to expand your team easily and painlessly by employing extra nursing time.

The FPC will reimburse 70% of ancillary staff salaries up to 72 hours per partner. A nurse working full time takes only half of that allowance, and though the practice must find 30% of the salary, some of that cost will be offset by additional fee-for-service items that will get done by the nurse. It is remarkable that the average number of ancillary staff employed by GPs under this scheme has stuck at just over one whole time equivalent per GP for the past 10 years, and 90% of these are receptionists.

GETTING AGREEMENT IN THE TEAM

Life will be easier if all in your practice agree on a policy of anticipatory care. Some will be keener than others, so the nurse or doctor who takes or is given responsibility for this preventive work must become a facilitator for others in the team. How do you motivate people to become interested in what they may see as an unrewarding area of care, with outcomes that seem undramatic and remote? Some health workers will never be interested and it may be better for them to say so and opt out; that is one option for your team discussions.

Your local health education officer should have some ideas about persuasive literature, films and posters for your colleagues, and you may even have one who is employed especially to help the primary health care team begin screening programmes to prevent heart disease and stroke, as we do in south Birmingham. Get along a charismatic speaker to address your team: the local heart specialist, a health education officer, a dietician, a physiotherapist or someone from a practice who already has such a system going. One option may be to screen the practice staff as a pilot project, if nobody minds other people knowing their business.

Of course, we are grateful for centrally produced health propaganda material of all kinds, particularly for television programmes, which at their best provide excellent material for personal and group discussion; but the most successful central material succeeds not because of its slick technicoloured production, but because it achieves by illusion a reality we already have in our own hands: the feeling of shared personal experience, involvement, and responsibility. Your own local data, the anecdotal experience of your own team, your own audit of your own work, are far more exciting to your team and your patients than anything you can get from the Health Education Council, important though it is. Some members of the team may be slow learners, but don't be too quick to dismiss them; perhaps they are merely sceptical of innovators who have yet to prove they can hold the new ground they are so keen to occupy. It is surprising how much attitudes change once people start discussing their own data rather than national statistics.

Getting started

It is easier to begin if you start where most of your team want to start.

Planned anticipatory care can begin anywhere; shaping up the care of known hypertensives or diabetics, sorting out your cervical smears' programme, or systematically doing something about smoking in your chronic coughers and wheezers. In every case the problems and their solutions will eventually appear essentially the same, and the measured, self-critical approach needed for one kind of anticipatory care will open everyone's eyes to similar opportunities in other fields. Most teams are happier starting with 'disease' groups like diabetics and hypertensives, rather than 'risk' groups like smokers, the obese, or heavy drinkers, but teams should start wherever their interests lie.

Don't look too far over the edge

It is also easier to begin if you don't worry too much about where it is all going to end. The destination will be the same whatever the entry point, because about half of all early deaths are from arterial disease, and these are concentrated in the least healthy groups, however defined: the diabetics, the hypertensives, the smokers, the obese, and the heavy drinkers. Looking too hard at the destination may easily daunt your team, and should be encouraged only if you are all confident that resources will one day be expanded to cope with it. There is no way practice teams as presently composed can complete the huge undertaking implied by all the chapters in this book.

Using data from the Royal College of General Practitioners' (RCGP) second national morbidity survey, Robson[1] showed that only to record blood pressure once every 5 years in people aged 45–64, and follow-up the borderline and hypertensive patients once a year, would require general practitioners (or other primary health workers) to undertake 286 per 1000 more consultations a year, over and above the 636 per 1000 now done in this age-group. This would represent a 45% increase in workload, if done with present practice organisation.

The size of your initial options

We gave you some figures in Chapter 2 which should help you to decide where to start.

Your smallest, most easily manageable, and highest risk group for coronary disease and stroke, is diabetics. They should be about 2% of your registered population, of whom half are likely to be known and half could be found by a programme of energetic case-finding concentrated on the elderly, the obese, and those with a family history of diabetes. Your local hospital diabetologist is likely to be interested and grateful if you seriously propose to take some of the routine work off his hands, and he may even offer you help from a specialist nurse and a dietician.

A larger option is hypertensives above the line for mandatory treatment at about 175/105mmHg, about 7% of your registered population, which will rise to about 10% if you add the people below this threshold with evidence of arterial damage. Again, about half of these will already be known, but half of them will be either poorly controlled or unknown. The latter half has to be found by systematic case-finding.

Bigger still is the army of smokers, 30–50% of your population depending on its social class composition. At least three-quarters of smokers probably have no indication of their smoking habits in your records, and few of those who do will have any account of efforts to help them stop.

Largest of all, 80% of your adult population will have abnormal cholesterol values which put them at risk for coronary heart disease. If you tackle them, you are really taking on the whole population.

One step at a time.

REFERENCE

1 Robson J. Bridging the expectation-delivery gap: can it be left to chance? *The Medical Annual: the year book of general practice* (eds Dereira Gray DJ, Dereira Gray J). Bristol: Wright, 1986.

Chapter 11
FINDING THE SMOKERS AND STOPPING THEM SMOKING

WHO SMOKES?

The simplest way is to ask, but though that seems too obvious to need discussion, a random sample of your records will probably reveal an alarming lack of information about smoking habits. Audits by training practices good enough to measure their own failings have shown that smoking habits are recorded in only about 15% of the records of men aged 35–64. Given that roughly two-thirds of the practice list are likely to attend at least once every year, and more than four-fifths attend at least once every 5 years, you have access to this information if you organise to obtain it. Here are some steps you can take to improve recorded information in your practice:

Step 1. At your next practice meeting, *discuss with everyone who sees patients the importance of recording smoking habits in the records*. It is important for nurses and doctors to ask about smoking, not only in order to permit categorisation of risk, but also because by implication this alerts patients to the risks they are running by smoking. It leads naturally to a discussion about smoking cessation, which is a vital beginning to preventive work.

Don't forget that community nurses and health visitors will be able to find out about their clients' smoking habits, perhaps with more accuracy and ease than the surgery-based staff. If they have access to your patients' records, and if they have accepted the idea of entering their information in them (an even bigger 'if'), they can make your information base more complete.

Step 2. *Decide where you are going to record smoking information* (Chapter 10 discusses some of the possibilities). If everybody uses the same method it is easier to retrieve the information. There may be some advantage in marking the outside of the notes, for again it makes patients aware of the importance attached to their smoking habits, and acts as a reminder for them at each consultation.

You should also decide how to indicate that a patient has stopped smoking. This has two effects: first, it can give patients a sense of achievement to see that they are no longer 'marked' as smokers, and second, it makes it easier to monitor progress with smoking cessation in your practice, simply by looking at the notes and counting your successes.

Step 3. *Think in terms of households rather than individuals.* This may be easier if all the notes relating to a family are filed together; easy with Lloyd-George (which can be fitted into an outer envelope), difficult with A4 (which are too bulky for any envelope; lacing with extra-long treasury tags is the cumbersome solution adopted in Glyncorrwg). When patients bring children to the surgery with coughs and colds, that's an opportunity to ask whether parents smoke. Indeed, the effect that a smoke-filled room has on a child's upper respiratory tract makes the question obligatory rather than optional. It's also worth asking children if they smoke.

Finding out about family smoking habits is essential for planning stopping strategies. Will one family member quit while others still smoke?

At what age should we stop? Risk of cardiovascular disease in people over the age of 65 who smoke cigarettes is increased, but much less than in younger age-groups. Given that smoking habits are by this time deeply ingrained, it's unlikely that any smoking cessation strategies will be effective if the patient's motive is to live longer and enjoy life. However, if there is *chronic obstructive airways disease* (COAD) causing breathlessness, or leg pain from obstructed arteries (intermittent claudication), then stopping smoking may relieve symptoms, or at least prevent further deterioration. If grandparents live with children and grandchildren, concern for their health may provide a motive for change. In general, however, you need to be much more selective in your approach to older smokers, with a greater readiness to take no for an answer.

Step 4. *Interviewing all new patients who sign on in your practice* serves many useful purposes. An interview allows patient and practitioner to get to know each other, and you can discover much about your patients' lifestyles while making a summarised history on the lines discussed in the last chapter. Inviting all new patients for a health check with nurse or doctor when they first join the practice gives everyone a sound base on which to plan further care.

Step 5. *Build audit into your strategy*. Try to agree as a team that after a certain period of time (say 3 months) when you have all been finding out and recording who smokes and how much, a random sample of notes will be drawn from the shelves and the proportion of patients whose smoking habits are recorded will be measured and compared with the figure before the start of your campaign.

You should all be doing better and this may act as a pat on the back for everyone, and inspire greater efforts. If the results are not so good it's an opportunity to ask why, and discuss your difficulties. Repeat this audit at 6 months, then annually. Not only is it interesting to know how well you are doing, but it will remind everyone to continue to ask patients about smoking habits.

Step 6. *Be ready to change your strategy if you find it doesn't work*. For example, you may discover that doctors have too little time with patients to undertake health teaching or screening. The team may prefer to delegate organised screening to a nurse, or to one of the clerical staff; after all, any honest and friendly person should be able to tackle smoking problems providing they are given access to patients, time for discussion, and some of the abundant literature available on the effects of smoking and techniques for stopping. On the other hand everyone might want to lengthen their consultation times to include more health teaching.

Here is a graphic summary of our steps to finding out who smokes:

ASK
MAKE A RECORD
ORGANISE A SEARCH
MEET THE NEWCOMERS
ASK THE FAMILY
SEE HOW WELL YOU'RE DOING
BE ADAPTABLE

QUITTING AND CUTTING DOWN – HOW CAN THEY DO IT?

In this chapter we list various methods which have been tried, and give you some idea of costs and likely success. It's important to find out what is available in your area and to keep a resource book of relevant addresses and telephone numbers available to all staff.

We begin where you will usually have to begin, in a one-to-one consultation with your patient.

Individual counselling

You may remember from Chapter 4 that if smokers are simply advised to stop and given a leaflet by their GP about the effects of smoking, 5% will quit for a year or more. This is evidence that patients are receptive to health advice given to them by their doctors (just advising to quit and handing over a leaflet can hardly be called a 'hard sell'), but only just. Whatever you do, you won't get big, quick, and easy results; it's not like treating pneumonia with penicillin, or asthma with a nebuliser. The best that even very intensive antismoking clinics have achieved is about 30% fewer smokers at follow-up after a year, and this was with selected groups at high risk and therefore with high motivation.

Insufficient research has been done on the effectiveness of nurses as health educators, though there is growing evidence that they can make a significant impact on behaviours affecting the control of hypertension. A recent project at Birmingham University, for example, found that a nurse caring for a group of hypertensive patients persuaded many of them to lose weight and give up or cut down on smoking with the result that a significant number of patients also cut down or were able to give up medication.

Give me one good reason . . .

For any education to be successful, the pupil must first be motivated to learn. In school, the motivation may be to pass exams or get a good job. However, much teaching about health starts not with motivation of the patients, but with the eagerness of teachers to impart what they know. Chapter 4 indicated that the sections of the population most likely to be well informed about health matters (social classes I and II, especially doctors) have been quick to cut down or give up cigarette smoking. Giving information about future health risk may motivate people who can understand the statistics and apply them to their own future. Evidence from behavioural scientists suggests that many less educated patients appear to have little interest in their future, and statistics have little meaning or relevance for them.

We think this is a defeatist argument. Of course statistics are meaningless if you don't have O-level maths, or if experience has taught you that statistics are more often used to confuse and mislead than to enlighten you; and planning for the future may appear futile for people who don't realistically expect to have one. For young people particularly, risk-taking, whether with motorbikes, cigarettes, alcohol, joining the army, or taking a chance without contraception, may all appear to make more immediate sense than letting your life be ruled by relatively elderly doctors and nurses who wag their fingers and know better.

However that may be, most patients in most practices are in social classes IIIb, IV, and V: manual workers with little academic education, but often better informed about the world they live in than most professionals. They are just as capable of learning, understanding, and valuing their own lives as social classes I, II, and IIIa, providing they are approached with respect, in their own language, and in terms of their own experience. The skills required for this have to be learned, for the most part on the job rather than from books.

Here is an example of what we mean:

Health educator: Have you ever thought of giving up smoking?

Client (42-year-old man, who had a myocardial infarction aged 38): Well I did once give up after my heart attack, and I didn't smoke for 3 years, but then about a year ago my uncle died of a heart attack and I had to make all the arrangements for him. It was a worrying time, you know, and I started thinking that maybe I'd die of a heart attack, too. As well as that I'd lost my job through illness and, well, you know what it's like getting jobs these days, so with the worry of it all I started smoking again. I'd like to give up because I know it costs a lot. The wife doesn't smoke and she'd like me to stop.

This is a particularly dramatic story (and a true one) of a most unfortunate man. He is potentially motivated to stop smoking, but will need support to succeed. The greatest help you could give him, of course, would be to get him a job, but failing that you can help him to understand that much of his life is still in his own hands, certainly as far as smoking and the risk of another heart attack is concerned. It's easy to see, though, that to give this information in a condescending or judgemental way will achieve little. Here is a worried man, who needs help not only with stopping smoking but to cope with his troubles. He needs support which will 'accentuate the positive'. He can give up (he's done it before), he can cut down his risk of another heart attack (he knows smoking's bad for him), he can save money, and he can please his wife.

If you let them, your patients will tell you their potential motivation for quitting. It may be illogical, funny or trivial, but it's that individual motive which will ensure success.

Believe me . . .

Most people have firm ideas about what may make them ill, cure them, or affect their health, and though such ideas are seldom accurate, they are influential.

> I smoke about 15 a day, I suppose, but sometimes it can be more because we both smoke and the kids too and we all have cigarettes in the house. Isn't it true that it's only dangerous smoking more than 20 a day? Someone at work told me that. Mind you, our Wayne, he's 15, he told me that at school they've had lessons about smoking and it's really very dangerous no matter how many you smoke. Still it hasn't stopped him so it can't be that bad, can it? (45-year-old woman.)

Health teaching is more likely to be effective if it reinforces correct health beliefs than if it corrects inaccurate ones. This lady has plenty of information about smoking, some accurate, some not. Basing your teaching on what she has told you ('Wayne is quite right' . . . rather than just 'there is no safe dose of cigarette smoke') will make more sense to her and be easier to remember. There is convincing evidence that people who are poorly educated and socio-economically disadvantaged tend to have a fatalistic attitude to health. These people are most likely to smoke cigarettes and to die early from smoking-related diseases. In finding out what your patients' health beliefs are and tailoring your support, information and advice accordingly, you will, perhaps surprisingly, be most influential with those patients whose need for information is greatest.

Let me tell you . . .

However much or little time you feel you can give to health education it is worth while having a structure for your teaching so that your work will be as effective as possible.

The next step is to give information about the effects of smoking and how to stop. What exactly you say will depend on your patients' individual need to know, and which method you and they think most likely to help them stop.

There are some ways of conveying information which are more likely to help your patient remember what you have said. Here are some tips:

THE GOLDEN RULES

- Be sure of your facts before you start.
- Have information you are likely to need at hand, such as addresses, health education booklets, diagrams.
- Be warm and supportive rather than punitive.
- Use language which your patient understands, short words and short sentences.
- Use pictures and drawings if this will help explanation.
- Start giving advice early in the consultation.
- Relate the information you give to the patient's own beliefs about health.
- Give booklets to reinforce your advice.
- Repeat important information, and get the patient to repeat it back to you.
- Remember to include the whole family in quitting strategies; this may mean another consultation with a couple or family group.
- Remember you are negotiating a voluntary contract: don't overdo your pressure on the patient.
- Try to conclude by agreeing a specific goal.
- Always arrange for a follow-up visit to go over your advice again and check on progress

GIVING UP

It's difficult to give up smoking; the number of people who fail testifies to this. Still, more than 8 million people in Britain have done it! Many methods have been tried from yoga through acupuncture to nicotine chewing-gum. The number of successful dodges worked out by patients themselves is extraordinary, and far too long to be listed here. Get several copies of the West Midlands Health Authority pamphlet if you can (see p. 121); it will help you, and stimulate your patients' imagination and confidence if you lend them a copy.

What you feel able to do depends on the time you have available and the skills of your practice staff. It's worth thinking seriously about employment of an extra person to concentrate on this job alone; there would be enough work to justify this even in quite a small group practice, with perhaps 4–5000 patients. The job definition (nominal and real) could perhaps be discussed with an imaginative and approachable FPC administrator, to see if it could be made to fit one of the reimbursable categories.

The GUS package

A landmark in British health education was the mass release by the Health Education Council in 1982 of the Give Up Smoking (GUS) package, a set of propaganda material for use by GPs. Its central feature is a small pamphlet (Fig. 11/1).

The idea is that the GP completes it just like an ordinary prescription, and hands it as personalised advice to the patient. This has proved more popular with GPs than any other single educational tool. It is still available free from the Health Educational Council.

Other self-help pamphlets and books

(This and the following six sections are taken (by permission) from the West Midlands Health Authority booklet *Quit Smoking*.)

The large majority of people who give up smoking do it on their own. Pamphlets and books can be a great help, but are not always easy to find. The format of most of them is the same: many facts about smoking and the damage it does, charts,

SURNAME
Mr./Mrs./Miss

Age if under 12 years

yrs. mths.

Initials and one full forename

Address

Pharmacy Stamp

Pharmacist's pack & quantity endorsement	No. of days treatment NB Ensure dose is stated	NP	*Pricing Office use only*

Give up Smoking!

Signature of Doctor

Date

For pharmacist No. of Prescns. on form

IMPORTANT: Read notes overleaf before going to the pharmacy.

Form FP1 (Rev. 78)

Fig. 11/1 GUS prescription form (*courtesy Health Education Council*) tables, guides and quizzes so that potential ex-smokers can monitor their progress, cash savings, and effect on weight. They contain practical advice on how to give up, how others gave up and answers to the most frequently asked questions about smoking and giving up. Often well-known personalities, especially sports people, are used to get the message across. Also included are exercise routines, calorie-counter charts, and a lot of encouragement.

SEVEN TYPES OF SMOKER

People smoke for different reasons and recognising the type you are dealing with is helpful. Russell[1] has suggested that there are seven basic types of smoker:

1 *Psychosocial smokers* smoke in a social situation and use smoking as a crutch to boost their confidence.
Advice: avoid the places where they most feel the urge to smoke. It won't be for ever.
2 *Sensory smokers* gain great satisfaction from the feel of a cigarette in the mouth or fingers.
Advice: get something to keep in their hands or mouth, for example worry beads, a dummy cigarette, even a pen or pencil.
3 *Indulgent smokers* do it for the actual pleasure of smoking or to heighten enjoyment of an already pleasurable moment.
Advice: reward themselves in some other way.
4 *Sedative smokers* use it as a comfort in the face of unpleasant feelings or to relieve tension.
Advice: relax some other way, for example a hot bath, breathing exercises, or a walk.
5 *Stimulative smokers* use it to help concentration and thinking, to ease tiredness or overcome boredom and monotony.
Advice: find something else that interests them and helps get them in the right frame of mind for work.
6 *Addictive smokers* do it to avoid the withdrawal symptoms of stopping.
Advice: use nicotine gum (see below). If their will power is strong enough the problem will pass, though it may take time.

7 *Automatic smokers* light cigarettes without even knowing it. *Advice*: hide cigarettes or avoid situations associated with smoking.

Some smokers don't fit any of these categories and need a mixture of ways to give up.

SEVEN GOOD WAYS TO STOP

1 *Stop dead – shock treatment.*
2 *Rapid smoking – smoke yourself sick.* They smoke two, three, or four times as many cigarettes as usual of a higher tar brand, with as little time as possible between cigarettes. In the end they can't tolerate another.
3 *Miser.* Save the money they would otherwise spend and use it for something worth while.
4 *Stop for the duration* of some suitable difficulty: a pregnancy, an attack of bronchitis, a cold or sore throat, or a child's respiratory illness.
5 *Estrangement.* Disrupt the smoking habit by changing to something unusual, for example smoking with the left hand instead of the right, or changing brands.
6 *Gradual giving up.* Sounds easy, but usually increasingly difficult as they approach the last cigarette.
7 *Bereavement.* Death from smoking is very common; in the family, among friends and workmates, even among celebrities, who are beginning to be a little more open about causes of death. It's a good time for stopping.

QUIT-SMOKING AIDS

There is no one cure for everyone, but all of these are successful in some people, and are obtainable from chemists.

CHEMICAL AIDS

Astringent aids, such as dilute silver nitrate solution, produce a foul taste in the mouth if mixed with tobacco smoke. The effects last 1–4 hours and mouthwashes must be repeated several times.

Tablets, lozenges and capsules are generally based on lobeline, which is supposed to give the satisfaction of nicotine without the harmful effects. There is no evidence that this is true, but like other harmless placebos, it is often effective.

NICOTINE CHEWING GUM (Nicorette)

Some practitioners believe this is an excellent method to stop smoking and have good results. Unfortunately it is not available through the NHS and it is expensive, though a little less so than cigarettes. This is a pity, because it means that patients who use it lose the considerable incentive of watching their piggy bank swell up as their smoking goes down.

With Nicorette, the craving for nicotine is satisfied by absorbing it through the mucous membranes of the cheek. Gum containing nicotine is chewed, and then held between the gum and cheek for as long as is needed. This is done each time the ex-smoker craves for a cigarette. It comes in two strengths, 2mg and 4mg, the latter is only needed for very heavy smokers, around 30 a day or more.

The disadvantage of Nicorette is that it is possible to become addicted to the gum itself. If seems that nicotine chewing-gum is most effective when the patient attends for group or individual counselling as well as using the gum. For more information you should contact the makers of the gum, Lundbeck, or Dr Chris Steele, a Manchester GP who runs excellent stop smoking groups and advocates the use of Nicorette gum (see p. 233 for addresses).

PSYCHOLOGICAL AIDS

There are about 50 smoking withdrawal clinics spread unevenly over Britain, mostly run by district health authorities (DHAs). On average they have a 10–20% success rate at follow-up after one year, usually among fairly heavy smokers. Few new clinics seem to be opening. It's worth asking your HA whether there is one in your locality.

Self-help groups are not quite so thin on the ground. *The Organiser's Handbook for Occupational Quit-smoking Programmes* by Robert East and Wendy Morton (p. 121), is particularly useful for anyone trying to start a group.

Hypnosis is effective for some people when done by a real

expert, but only about one person in three is hypnotisable. Charges are usually high, but this may help to ensure subsequent compliance ('a pity to waste all that money').

MECHANICAL AIDS

MD4 filters come in packs of 4. You are supposed to use each filter for only 2 weeks, and each filters out a progressively higher proportion of the tar and nicotine in cigarette smoke. After 8 weeks the user is supposed to have been weaned off cigarettes. The disgusting state of the filters may have an educational effect.

Targuard filters are claimed to reduce the level of tar, but (unlike MD4) the makers do not claim that they help people to give up.

Apal dummy cigarettes look and feel like a cigarette and contain mint-flavoured crystals which are claimed to 'take away the craving to smoke'.

LOW-TAR AND HERBAL CIGARETTES

The harmful effects of cigarette smoking, and to a much smaller extent cigar and pipe smoking, probably arise from 3 more or less independent sources: tar, carbon monoxide, and nicotine.

The lung cancer promoting factor is probably the tar; lung cancer and perhaps bronchitis and emphysema risks may be less with low-tar brands and with filters, though there is no really good evidence of this. There is no reason why low-tar brands should give any protection against the effects of smoking on the heart and arteries, and no evidence that they do this.

Even herbal cigarettes release a variable amount of tar and carbon monoxide, probably with harmful effects on the heart. Even at best they still maintain the smoking habit.

People who have never smoked cigarettes rarely inhale cigar or pipe smoke, but ex-cigarette smokers nearly always do so, whether they realise it or not; so cigars and lit pipes are not a good alternative for cigarette smokers. Unlit pipes, on the other hand, can be very useful, giving all the appearance of wisdom and maturity, without the folly of real smoking.

USEFUL BOOKS AND LEAFLETS FOR QUIT-SMOKING WORK

The GUS package and much other antismoking material is available free from the Health Education Council, 78 New Oxford Street, London WC1A 1AH.

Public Relations Division, West Midlands Regional Health Authority, Arthur Thomson House, 146 Hagley Road, Birmingham B16 9PA issue the following pamphlets (1983):

The People Say How They Gave Up Smoking.

Quit Smoking: A Summary of Smoking Cessation Techniques.

Robert East and Bridget Towers, Kingston Polytechnic, Health Education Research Team, Penrhyn Road, Kingston-upon-Thames KT1 2EE have written (1979):

No Smoke: A Psychologically Based Manual of Information and Self-applied Exercises for Use in Giving Up Smoking.

Robert East and Wendy Moreton, same address, (1980):

Organiser's Handbook for Occupational Quit-smoking Programmes.

A range of posters and other useful materials is available from the same address.

Royal College of Physicians of London, Pitman Medical (1977):

Smoking or Health; Third Report of the RCP.

Peter Taylor, The Bodley Head (1984):

Smoke Ring: The Politics of Tobacco.

Badges ('I'm quitting', 'Submerge the urge', and 'No smoke') are available from Better Badges, 286 Portobello Road, London W10.

REFERENCE

1 Russell M, Peto J, Patel U. Classification of smokers by factorial structure of motives. *Journal of the Royal Statistical Society* 1974;**137**:313.

Chapter 12
FINDING HIGH BLOOD PRESSURE

HOW HIGH IS 'HIGH'?

Clinical trials which have tested the effects, positive and negative, of treating blood pressure at different levels have been discussed in Chapter 5. Here we summarise our criteria for management of hypertension by controlling other risk factors only, or together with antihypertensive medication, in people without evidence of organ damage.

The three box system

For practical purposes, we need not one but two thresholds: one to define the group who are likely to gain more than they will lose from treatment with antihypertensive drugs, even if they show no evidence of organ damage and have no symptoms; and a lower one to define people whose blood pressures are high enough to require observation but not medication, who may benefit from measures to reduce blood pressure other than drugs, and will certainly benefit from control of other risk factors. This is what Dr John Coope, who invented it, called a 'three box system'; Box One for normal blood pressure, Box Two for borderline high blood pressure, and Box Three for blood pressure high enough to need medication.

Why three?

Why do we need Box Two, the observation group? First,

because blood pressure rises with age, and more rapidly at higher pressures. Within a screened population all of whose pressures are known, virtually all new hypertensives who may appear during a 5-year span will come from this group. Second, because although on present evidence treatment with antihypertensive drugs is seldom justified below a pressure of 175/105mmHg, other measures to reduce risk, above all control of cigarette smoking, should be offered to this group at higher risk and therefore potentially more motivated than the general population. Finally, they may be a target group for other measures to reduce blood pressure.

We suggest that Box Two should be defined as those with pressures of 150/90–174/104mmHg. There are more than three times as many of these borderline hypertensives as there are in Box Three, the mandatory treatment group above the threshold 175/105mmHg. We think they need review at least once a year, in contrast to the 'normotensives' in Box One, who need to be reviewed only once every five years.

To summarise:

BOX ONE

Mean of 3 systolic pressures	<150	Measure and act on smoking and obesity Re-measure BP in 5 years
or		
Mean of 3 diastolic pressures	<90	

BOX TWO

Mean of 3 systolic pressures	150–174	Measure and act on smoking, obesity and high blood cholesterol Re-measure BP annually
or		
Mean of 3 diastolic pressures	90–104	

BOX THREE

Mean of 3 systolic pressures	175+	Measure and act on smoking, obesity, high cholesterol; start antihypertensive drugs; review every 3 months, or less if uncontrolled
or		
Mean of 3 diastolic pressures	105+	

Patients with evidence of arterial or organ damage, or with diabetes, should be treated with antihypertensive drugs from a threshold of 150/90. The treatment target for most patients will be below this threshold.

GETTING ORGANISED

As always, start with the records: see what information you already have, and organise it in such a way that whenever a patient consults, you can see what additional information is needed (Chapter 10). Then:

- *Use your age sex register to estimate the size of the task.* You will have to decide what age-groups to tackle; inclusion of older people will give you more people in urgent need of treatment, on the other hand the small number of cases of severe hypertension in relatively young people under 40 is particularly important to find, because of the much greater potential saving of life. In Glyncorrwg we screened everyone between 20 and 64, and went on to do all the elderly later; we should probably have done better to have started at 35 and included everyone up to 70 from the start. Your rate of recruitment of new cases will depend on your consultation rate, which is likely to be 60–75% of the list each year (less in young men), and about 90% over 5 years.
- *Take a 10% random sample from the records in the age-group you have agreed on*: how many patients have had a blood pressure recorded during the last 5 years? How many have no record of blood pressure at all? How many patients have evidence of known hypertension? How many of these still seem to be having treatment? How many have not been seen for 6 months, or for a year or more? How many seem to have been started on treatment on wrong or doubtful criteria?
- *By the same method of random sampling, use your file of oral contraception claim forms (FP1001) to identify women on the pill.* Are blood pressures being recorded efficiently? Are there any with pressures already over the threshold 150/90 whose rise in pressure has been ignored?

You are sure to find that your data is very incomplete. Practices which have been through this process generally find that one-third or less of their adult patients have had any measurement of blood pressure recorded during the previous 5 years, and no practice we know of has recorded more than 50% at this stage. You will probably find some severe hypertensives who have not been checked for a year or two, and others for whom it is unclear from their records whether they ever started medication. Another possible source of data is your repeat prescribing list, though this is sometimes ambiguous because diuretics are used both as antihypertensive drugs, and as treatment for heart failure and oedema.

Where data is incomplete or patients have not been followed up, mark the records as suggested in Chapter 10 to alert the next user. You will find a few severe hypertensives (pre-treatment diastolic pressures 120+) who should be actively sought out by letter or telephone call, because these people are at high risk. By starting treatment in the past, you have made yourself legally responsible for continued follow-up.

Planning ahead

Once you have this data from your 10% random sample, you are in a position to give your whole team some idea of what they are taking on, and choices can be made about what is to be done, who is going to do it, who it is to be done to, how fast, and in what order of priority. The evidence you will find of potentially dangerous gaps will help your staff to see that reform is necessary, urgent, and potentially satisfying.

For example, in the light of the evidence of future workload, you may decide to widen or reduce the age-range of your programme; to tidy up the management of your known but perhaps somewhat neglected hypertensives, by getting people back under regular monitoring if they seem really to need treatment, or seeing how they get on without medication if the original indications seem doubtful; or you may want to reach decisions about whether to set up a separate clinic for your hypertensives.

We now know that the proportion of severe hypertensives

varies between populations, mainly according to their social class; you can expect up to one-third more cases in an area with many unskilled, semiskilled, or unemployed workers. Even so, the potential numbers are broadly predictable; from experience at Glyncorrwg, in an average list of 2200 we would expect you to find 150 people at most requiring antihypertensive medication, using Box Three criteria plus all diabetics or people with evidence of arterial or organ damage, with mean blood pressure >150/90.

Records and recall systems
This has been fully discussed in Chapter 10.

PEOPLE

Who is going to do the work?

In Handsworth, with a practice list of 7500 the bulk of the hypertension screening and treatment is carried out by nurses. For four mornings a week a nurse is employed whose only job is to measure blood pressure, and monitor blood pressure treatment. She works closely with one of the GPs who sees patients causing her concern, or who she thinks should begin drug treatment. All patients who are found by anyone in the practice to have an initially high blood pressure reading can be referred to 'the hypertensive nurse' (as she has unfortunately come to be called) for subsequent readings. Patients who have been found to have borderline blood pressures (<170/100) who need annual reviews are recalled to see our generalist practice nurse, who undertakes such blood pressure checks for half a morning a week.

The system in Glyncorrwg reflects the much smaller size of the practice (1700). Both the two part-time practice nurses, the principal GP and the trainee are all supposed to look out for people whose BP measurements are outstanding (we enter the next year they are due on a sticker inside the front flap of the A4). Nearly all measurements are done by nurses, who check weight and smoking at the same time. First high readings are always followed up by at least two further readings, and in most cases patients with borderline pressures are taught how to use an electronic sphygmomanometer, take it home on loan, and return with 28 home readings. We base our eventual decision to use or withhold antihypertensive medication on the average of all 28 readings. We hold an evening hypertension clinic once a fortnight, at which about two-thirds of the follow-up patients are seen only by the nurse, and the rest see both the nurse and the doctor. We aim to see all patients on medication once every three months, sooner if their control is poor.

A recent research project at Birmingham University[1] demonstrated how well a nurse could measure blood pressure, initiate and monitor drug treatment according to an agreed protocol, and also encourage patients to lose weight and stop smoking. Nurses are particularly good at using protocols sensibly as well as being empathetic and patient teachers. The Cumberlege review of community nursing (1986) has recommended easier access to nurses by patients, so any practice planning to attach health authority nurses rather than employ its own should feel on solid ground in requesting more nursing hours.

Make use of that policy, and of nurses' under-used talents, to enhance your screening and treatment programmes. How much clerical help do you need? If you have one receptionist/clerk who is able to take responsibility for the organisation of your screening, then the system will probably work better, in the same way as it will with one nurse and one doctor who take responsibility for implementing policy. However, such specialisation is possible only in fairly large group practices, and one of us (JTH) thinks it is unnecessary and potentially harmful, by encouraging compartmentalised thinking. It is important to remember that any really effective structure you set up is likely to last several generations, and may not retain the flexibility and imagination of its pioneers.

A possible compromise is to involve all the doctors and most of the nurses in your programme, but give one doctor and one nurse the job of pushing the work forward (progress-chasing), mastering the large volume of new literature, and reporting it back to the team at your clinical meetings.

Delegation of work must at the very least be accompanied by

an explicit protocol for management, including simple criteria for referral back. At best it should include nurses and any other health workers in the team in regular clinical meetings, where audited local experience can be discussed and knowledge of new developments from the medical and nursing literature can be shared.

CASE-FINDING OR CALL-UP SCREENING?

Over a 5-year period a practice is likely to be consulted by 90% of its patients, so that a policy of opportunistic screening can in theory at least reach almost that proportion of the whole registered population. In practice it will certainly be less than this, because many patients consult for reasons such as high fever or in tears, which would invalidate any readings made at such times. A much more important source of default is simply that opportunist screening (case-finding) is rarely implemented in practice, until audit of randomly sampled records proves to all members of the team that despite their promises, everyone is carrying on pretty much as before.

Even if you decide to opt mainly for case-finding, you will probably need to supplement that with call-up screening for non-attenders after your first 5 years. In the Handsworth practice the main non-attenders were middle-aged men (42–55) and we now send for this group of men every 2 years for a full screening because they are such an important risk group.

Call-up screening allows you to decide in advance whom you want to attend, when, and what for. You can decide to invite husbands and wives together, which usually gets a better response, and sets the scene well for discussion of all risk factors. You can decide what your priorities are, both for screening and treatment, and more easily regulate your work load. However, it is costly in postage, and the yield rarely exceeds 60% response to the first letter. Many of the people at highest risk are likely to be non-respondents, though probably they would readily agree to a blood pressure check in the course of a consultation for some other purpose. Few GPs have in fact chosen the call-up strategy and stuck to it right through; the only one we know of is John Coope in Bollington, Cheshire. Chapter 10 tells you more about reorganising your records to enable you to plan efficient screening, whether you choose either of these methods, or more likely some combination of both.

You are aiming eventually to see all men aged 20–65 (see Chapter 3 for our reasoning) and women from the start of oral contraception or age 20, whichever is the sooner, to age 65. Obviously you want a gradual increase in your workload rather than a sudden onslaught which will immediately dishearten everyone, so go first for men (who have a higher risk because of their gender) aged 35–50, and widen your target population as you are able. Be sure to allow enough time not only to do your measurements of blood pressure, weight, height, and smoking, but also to explain the results to the patients. A realistic plan would be to send for 20 patients, expecting 15 to turn up, for one 2-hour session serviced by a doctor, a nurse, and a receptionist. You should allow another 30 minutes at each end for organisational work.

MEASURING BLOOD PRESSURE

As 90% of clinical decisions in management of high blood pressure depend on this measurement, obviously it is important to get it right. For many reasons, few doctors and even fewer nurses have ever been properly taught how to do this simple procedure. One of us (JTH) has just gone through 100 blood pressures reported in hospital correspondence; 90% of the systolic pressures and 85% of the diastolic pressures ended in a zero, which clearly means that most of the people taking the pressures were measuring them to the nearest 10mmHg. Which nearest? Nearest up, or nearest down? We don't know, but what a difference it makes. Nurses who have had to maintain half-hourly BP charts which no one ever seemed to look at will be familiar with blood pressures which start at 110/70 and stay there all day no matter what the patient is doing.

Why are BP measurements such a shambles? We can think of three reasons:

1 Blood pressure is a moving target, so people think they are more likely to hit it with a shotgun than a precision rifle. Since any one measurement is wildly unrepresentative of the true average pressure, why bother to measure accurately? The answer is, of course, *never* to base major clinical decisions on a single reading, but to obtain several readings, each as accurate as possible, and act on the mean.
2 Doctors order BP readings as they order TPR charts or daily electrolyte estimations; out of habit, ignoring the results. If no one ever acts on the information you record, you soon lose interest in its accuracy. Readings should not only be looked at, but used for audit of the work of the whole team.
3 Measuring BP is uncomfortable for the patient, as everyone who has ever been pregnant knows. Rapid deflation of the cuff quickly restores comfort to the patient, at the cost of false–low readings: a cruel kindness if that patient is left untreated and ends up with a stroke.

It's best to assume that the whole team, doctors included, need retraining in BP measurement.

An 8-Point checklist on measurement of blood pressure

1 *Make it an absolute rule that no one is ever started on anti-hypertensive medication without at least 3 BP readings*. These should be on separate days unless there is a true hypertensive emergency such as a neuroretinopathy, left ventricular failure, or transient cerebral ischaemic attack; even then, take 3 replicate readings. The average of these 3 readings is then the pretreatment pressure, an important figure to record in the summary chart.
2 *The patient should be sitting relaxed*. Standing and lying pressures are only useful if you are looking for postural hypotension, usually in diabetics or the elderly.
3 *The rubber bladder inside the cuff should be applied so that its mid-point lies over the brachial artery, on the inside of the biceps tendon, and it should be long enough to encircle the arm*. Insist on having a full set of cuffs (small for children, adult, large adult, and extra-large adult) with range lines so

that you can tell straightaway if you're applying the wrong cuff. These are available from both Accoson and Baumanometer. The lower edge of the cuff should be far enough above the elbow crease to be clear of the stethoscope diaphragm; this often means removing sleeves rather than rolling them up.

4 *The patient's arm should be resting comfortably on a table, so that the cuff is level with the heart.* Always use the same arm; it doesn't matter which, but the same.

5 *Use a mercury sphygmomanometer* recording up to 300mmHg, with the glass tube and the rubber bulb filter *cleaned at least once every 6 months*, and the valve washers changed at least once a year. As soon as rubber tubing shows little cracks it should be replaced. The glass must be vertical and at roughly eye level. *Electronic machines are not yet reliable* enough for anything but home readings, and aneroid machines are not dependable.

6 Inflate the cuff until you are unable to hear sounds over the brachial artery, or feel a pulse at the wrist. Then *deflate slowly* at a steady rate of 3mm a second, roughly one 2mm division per heartbeat.

7 Record systolic pressure as the point at which the first regular sounds begin, to the nearest 2mm down. *Systolic pressure is easier to recognise and of greater prognostic value than diastolic pressure* (contrary to what most of us have been taught). Avoid categorising patients only by diastolic pressure; high systolic pressures are important, particularly in the elderly.

8 *Record diastolic pressure as the point at which regular sounds disappear* (phase 5). If the sounds never disappear, even when all clothing has been removed, use the point at which the sounds suddenly become muffled (phase 4) and note that you have done so. Phase 5 is now almost universally accepted as standard in the USA, and is rapidly becoming standard in the UK.

Some common reasons for false high blood pressure readings

The patient:

was *cold*,

had a *full bladder*,
had *rushed* to the surgery,
was *frightened*,
was *depressed*,
or had a *tense arm*.

The cuff was too short for a *fat arm*.
The mercury column was *tilted* backwards.

Some common reasons for false low blood pressure readings

- There was *tight clothing* around the upper arm.
- The cuff was deflated and the mercury *dropped too quickly*.
- You *pressed too hard* with your stethoscope over the brachial artery.

Your readings will be inaccurate if . . .

- Your sphygmomanometer is not well maintained, particularly if the glass is too dirty to see the level of the mercury clearly, or the valves are leaking.
- You forget what the systolic pressure was by the time you have got to the diastolic.
- You read only to the nearest 10mm.
- You guess that the pressure will be similar to the last one recorded.
- You record not what you actually heard, but what you think you ought to have heard.

BASELINE MEASUREMENTS AND INVESTIGATIONS

When you think you have found a Box One or Box Two hypertensive, other measurements, history, examinations, and investigations need to be done. They are required for three reasons:

- To evaluate other risks for coronary disease and stroke, chiefly smoking, obesity, and blood cholesterol.

- To establish baselines against which to evaluate later change. For example, unless you know whether ankle and foot pulses are present now, you cannot know later when they have been lost; unless you do an ECG now, you cannot know whether Q waves are new and significant, or old and caused by a bundle-branch block; unless you know what the PEFR is before treatment, you can't know if a low value later on has been caused by your treatment. In fact nearly all the routine investigations needed for good care of hypertensives are baselines of this kind.
- Finally, to search for causes of secondary hypertension. This function has been unrealistically over-emphasised in the past. Apart from checking oral contraception and a brief search for the delayed or absent femoral pulses of coarctation of the aorta, no other routine investigations for secondary hypertension are cost-effective at this stage, except in very young patients (under 30). Most of them will be found later, usually because response to treatment is anomalous. However, several of these rare causes should be detected from baseline measurements required for other reasons: for example, aldosterone-secreting tumours are usually revealed by a low plasma potassium level found on routine baseline measurement of potassium as a baseline for evaluating any fall in potassium following prolonged use of diuretics.

EXPLAINING TO PATIENTS AND THEIR FAMILIES

Explain as you go along what you are doing, and why you are doing it. At some point both patient and spouse should be seen together, to explain the nature of high blood pressure as a continuously distributed, rather unstable variable, and as a partially reversible risk factor, *not* a disease; and the nature of its treatment as a probably *permanent* change in lifestyle (smoking, eating, exercise, and perhaps regular pill-taking) requiring indefinite follow-up. Make copies of the relevant leaflets in Chapter 21 and use them to back up what you have said. You may be able to improve on them by modifying them to suit your local population.

SUGGESTED SEQUENCE FOR EARLY DATA COLLECTION

First (identification) visit

ASKING AND LISTENING

Smoking.

Family history of stroke, coronary disease, diabetes, and causes of death in parents and siblings.

Current symptoms, especially those attributed by the patient to hypertension.

Current medication, especially oral contraception and antidepressants.

MEASURING

ECG, PEFR, urine for glucose and protein, height, weight.

EXAMINING

Fundoscopy, heart for size and rhythm disorders, lungs for crackles, ankle and foot pulses.

INVESTIGATING

Sequestrene blood for *full blood count* (FBC); clotted blood for biochemical screen including potassium (must be centrifuged and partitioned if there will be more than 2 hours' delay before measurement) urea, creatinine, urate, and *gamma glutamyl transferase* (GGT); sequestrene blood for *glycosylated haemoglobin* (HbA1c) if BMI=35+ or there is a family history of diabetes.

Arrange repeat BP measurements on at least 2 more separate days.

Arrange fasting lipid profile.

Second visit

Review results of baseline measurements, especially lipid profile, renal function (urea and creatinine) and indicators for alcohol (MCV=95+, high triglyceride, raised GGT).

Take a diet history concentrating on fat and alcohol intake.

For smokers, find out how many times they have stopped or tried to stop, why they relapsed, what they already think and know about smoking and health.
Record current exercise at home and at work, past and potential future interests.

Are there any major problems at home or at work?
Ask specifically about sex function.

Third visit
Arrange if possible for the spouse to accompany the patient.
Discuss investigation results, negotiate a plan for control of other coronary and stroke risk factors.
Take a decision to:
review BP annually, or
teach patient or spouse to do home recordings and return in 2 weeks with 28 readings, or
initiate antihypertensive medication and return to follow-up clinic in 4 weeks.

A PROTOCOL FOR NURSES RUNNING A HYPERTENSION CLINIC

This is the protocol used at Glyncorrwg for many years; it is only a guide, and should be modified to suit your local requirements.

Blood pressure clinics are held every fortnight from 16.15 to 18.00. The clinic is run by a practice nurse with a doctor available for advice and referral.

Ascertainment, initial diagnostic work-up, and initiation of patient education and treatment are all done in ordinary sessions and should be completed before referral to the blood pressure clinic, which normally deals with people already stabilised on treatment and fairly well controlled.

The *aims* of the clinic are:

1 To check blood pressure, medication, body-weight, and current smoking in all treated hypertensives at least once every 3 months.
2 To control pressures below 160/90mmHg (good control), or 175/100mmHg (partial control).

3 To verify that patients understand their medication, and if not, explain it to them; and to enquire about any side-effects suspected by the patient.
4 To control Body Mass Index (metric weight divided by the square of metric height) below 30.0.
5 In patients who still smoke, to enquire about respiratory symptoms, and use these or other opportunities to re-open negotiations on stopping when the time seems right to do this.

Procedures

Whenever a new hypertensive patient is detected in the course of ordinary surgery sessions the patient's record will be marked with a *blue tab* on the spine, and the name and address will be noted and given to you. Before the next clinic you should enter the name, address, and telephone number, if any, on a card, which you should place in a *boxed card-index* containing all hypertensives known to the practice, grouped in clinic date order so that everyone should be seen not less than once every 3 months. At each clinic the cards filed for that session should be date-stamped, with a note on whether the patient attended or defaulted. No other information should go on this card, except for information which may help to improve contact. For example, note new telephone numbers, people who are house-bound and will need a visit from the doctor or community nurse, have special difficulties such as odd shifts, or can't sit in the waiting room because of phobic symptoms.

One week *before the clinic*, look through the group listed for it and ask the receptionist to extract these patients' records. Look at the last entry. If the patient has had a blood pressure check within the last 3 months and was well controlled, give them a new date 3 months ahead, enter this on the card, and put it back in the box at the appropriate date. If the patient seems to be housebound, ask the practice manager to give the visit either to one of the doctors or to a community nurse, whichever was responsible for the last entry. If the patient defaulted the last clinic, consider ringing him up or visiting him at home to find out what the difficulty is in attending. For all the others, send out a written invitation to attend the clinic, with an appointment time.

Frequent defaulters should be reminded by telephone, if they have one.

At the clinic start seeing patients as soon as they begin to arrive, usually 15 minutes or so before the doctor is due. Enter the date, and if the patient has defaulted or sent an apology, record this. Ask patients how they have been since their last clinic visit, and have a look at the last entry in their record to see if something new has happened since then. Ask the patient to show you his or her antihypertensive tablets, which should *always* be brought to the clinic, and check that they are being taken as recorded on the repeat prescription sheet. This is an opportunity to discuss any difficulties they have with the tablets, remembering to take them or possible side-effects.

Then measure and record the following data, both in the patient's record and on the encounter form:

Blood pressure. Use phase 5 (disappearance of sound) for diastolic pressure, and record to the nearest 2mmHg, with the mercury descending at a rate of roughly 2mm per pulse beat. Tell the patient the result.

Pulse rate. Count pulse over 15sec. and multiply by four.

Current smoking in cigarettes a day.

Weight in kilograms.

Peak expiratory flow rate (PEFR) if this was recorded at the last visit.

Ask every patient if, for *any* reason, they would like to see the doctor. The doctor will be seeing other non-hypertensive patients, but he or she will be under less pressure than you are and *all* patients who want to see the doctor should do so.

Refer patients to the doctor in the following circumstances:

If systolic pressure is over 160mmHg or diastolic pressure is over 90mmHg. Before referral, ask the patient why he or she thinks the blood pressure is poorly controlled, e.g. forgetting or lapsing medication, drinking more alcohol, worries at home, and check other medication with indomethacin or other anti-arthritic drugs, or oral contraception.

If pulse rate is less than 60.

If you think, and the patient agrees, that it would be useful to tackle smoking again and discussion with the doctor could help in this.

If you think, and the patient agrees, that it would be useful to tackle obesity again and discussion with the doctor could help in this.

If the patient has not seen a doctor for a year or more.

If you are worried for any reason about the patient.

On average, we expect about one-third of the patients to need referral to the doctor.

After the clinic discuss any interesting or difficult cases, and each defaulter, with the doctor. Decide on action to be taken in respect of each defaulter.

Once every 3 months:

Check that every record with a blue tab has a card in the boxed index, and

Check every card in the index to see that everyone in it has either been seen, or that arrangements are in hand for them to be seen.

This will take you an hour or two. If you need more time, raise this at the next practice staff meeting.

REFERENCE

1 Kenkre J, Drury VWM, Lancashire RJ. Nurse management of hypertension clinics in general practice assisted by a computer. *Family Practice* 1985;**2**:17.

If you want a more detailed account of high blood pressure and its management, you will find it in Julian Tudor Hart's *Hypertension*, published by Churchill Livingstone (2nd edition, 1987).

Chapter 13

CONTROLLING HIGH BLOOD PRESSURE

Towards the end of the last chapter we touched on the need to explain to patients and their families the nature of their problem.

How do patients feel about having high blood pressure? We have given you some of the evidence on this in Chapter 5: in general, patients believe that high blood pressure is a disease causing symptoms (mainly headache, flushing, palpitations and giddiness), and that 'hypertension' means tense nerves and a generally wrought-up state. Their views will be influenced by family members or friends who have had, or think they have had, high blood pressure. If a close relative has died of a stroke caused by high blood pressure, this may throw patients into a panic, fearing imminent death, particularly if they interpret their headaches or giddiness as early symptoms of such a disaster.

All these beliefs are wrong. High blood pressure, mild or severe, rarely causes symptoms, and patients whose high blood pressure is identified by routine screening (as will soon be the case for 90% of the cases you see in your practice, once you begin to apply the ideas in this book) are particularly unlikely to develop complications quickly. Providing the patient is not already gasping with left ventricular failure, and you have looked at the fundi and ruled out any retinal bleeds, even the highest pressures can be dealt with quietly, sensibly, and without panic. Hypertension is *not* the same as high nervous tension. Of course, fear raises blood pressure as long as it lasts, but it is rarely a cause of sustained high blood pressure, which is why tranquillisers are generally useless in its treatment. Though relaxation treatment probably does help at least some people with high blood pressure, feeling relaxed is not a safe guide to the state of blood pressure.

Unless these beliefs are corrected, as soon as patients stop having their headaches, flushes, giddinesses, palpitations and fears, they are likely to stop their treatment and default from follow-up. The key to good compliance is understanding, and the key to understanding is knowledge. If you don't tell them, how can they know, and if they don't know, how can they understand? If they believe high blood pressure is caused by tension and they are not tense, they will not believe their blood pressure can still be dangerously high.

Your aim is to give patients understandable information about the ways in which losing weight, stopping smoking, taking exercise and learning to relax may influence the risks of high blood pressure; not how they may influence the pressure, but how they may influence the risks. Smokers generally have slightly lower blood pressure than non-smokers, but they have enormously greater risks of heart disease, and somewhat higher risks of stroke.

IT ISN'T ALL PILLS

High blood pressure can be brought under control in several ways, only some of which involve drugs. It is true that blood pressures sustained at or above the threshold we recommend for mandatory treatment, about 175/105, can hardly ever be controlled without medication, but even then doses may be lower and the number of drugs fewer, if other contributory causes such as obesity and alcohol are tackled. And for the 75% or so of people with high blood pressure below this threshold, these non-drug measures are the only alternative to doing either nothing at all, or misusing drugs for a condition in which there is no evidence of net benefit from medication.

ACTION ON OTHER RISK FACTORS

There is no need to repeat here the detailed advice given in Chapters 4, 6, and 7, on the nature of other risk factors, and Chapters 11, 15, 16, and 17 on their control. Control of some of these will actually reduce blood pressure, though usually only by a small margin; but this is not the main point, the important thing is to reduce risks of coronary disease and stroke. It is essential not to allow the label 'hypertension' to justify inaction on other equally or even more important or more easily reversible risks which the patient may have.

Everyone with high blood pressure is at greater risk from coronary disease and stroke. Stroke risk can be reduced by about 50% by controlling high blood pressure below 150/90, but coronary risk has been almost unaffected by reduction of blood pressure in controlled trials comparing treated and untreated cases. Action on smoking is urgent and essential, because stopping smoking quickly reduces coronary risk by about 50%, and stroke risk rather less than this. It should therefore be given initial priority, though of course persistent smoking is *not* a reason for inaction on other risks, including the control of high blood pressure. Most people (with or without high blood pressure) have high blood cholesterol. Though useful action on this can be taken without measuring blood cholesterol, we think compliance with dieting is likely to be better if initial measurements are made (at least of total cholesterol, which doesn't need fasting blood), and if feedback is given by at least one or two further measurements after dieting has begun.

Relaxation

Teaching patients to relax can probably bring down blood pressure as effectively as drugs, in people with blood pressures in the range 150–174/90–104. Above these levels it may reduce the dosage of antihypertensive medication needed to control pressure, but is not sufficient on its own. We must re-emphasise that on present evidence, this and other behavioural treatments should not be regarded as safe and effective alternatives to antihypertensive drugs for people with blood pressures at and over 175/105.

Chandra Patel[1] has pioneered this treatment in the UK, and has found that learning physical and mental relaxation techniques has reduced moderately raised blood pressure for up to 2 years in carefully controlled trials. Dr Patel has taught her patients breathing exercises, deep muscle relaxation and meditation to produce relaxation. They have also been taught how to integrate these techniques with their everyday lives, and been made aware of the links between 'stress' and high blood pressure in at least some patients, though it certainly does not explain them all. The connection between 'stress' and heart disease is more uncertain, with conflicting results from research which by no means support the rather simple assumption that, for example, the stress of competitive sport does you good, while the stress of paying bills with money you don't have does you harm. Perhaps unhappiness or inability to relax are the factors involved, but again they may be important causes in some people but not in others.

If someone in your practice has a particular interest in learning about relaxation skills, it might be worth delegating that person to attend classes, which may be run by the local community psychiatric nurses, physiotherapists or a specialist yoga group. Alternatively consider asking a yoga teacher to come and teach relaxation to a group of patients (this was successful in the Handsworth practice). The educational work, making the links between stress and high blood pressure, can be done by one of the practice staff, before the relaxation session. It is easy to demonstrate the fall in blood pressure which occurs after relaxation therapy, by taking before and after readings, but remember that blood pressure high enough to need medication can rarely be controlled by this means alone.

Watch out for and treat depressed patients. They often have a raised blood pressure which will usually return to normal when their depression is treated or remits on its own. High blood pressure in depressed patients is often resistant to conventional antihypertensive drugs, which may make depression worse. In nearly all cases, the depression should be treated first, and the high blood pressure should not be tackled until depression has been controlled.

Alcohol

Taken regularly, too much alcohol is an important cause of high blood pressure. How much is too much? Present evidence suggests that 4 glasses of wine, 4 measures of spirits, or 2 pints of beer a day will not lead to a rise in blood pressure. These fairly small quantities of alcohol probably reduce the risk of coronary heart disease, not by an effect on blood pressure, but by an effect on blood fats. Starting from intakes twice this level (8 glasses of wine, 8 single measures of spirits, or 4 pints of beer), alcohol begins to raise blood pressure and to increase vascular risk, particularly the risk of stroke; and of course it may lead to addiction, liver damage, peripheral nerve damage, and obesity.

It is worth asking about alcohol intake in detail for three reasons. First, what seems reasonable to your patient may be a lot more than what is healthy. Second, patients are generally unaware of the links between alcohol and disease, particularly if their social behaviour is not grossly affected. There is a common assumption that alcohol cannot be doing physical harm if there is no obvious intoxication. In fact, cirrhosis of the liver occurs mainly in people who hold their liquor well, and the same is probably true of effects on blood pressure. Patients often respond surprisingly well to accurate information, particularly if it is backed up by evidence of physical effects (raised MCV, triglyceride, or GGT), and if reduced intake is rewarded by feedback of improved values.

The third reason is that patients may know they have a problem with heavy drinking, and welcome an opportunity to talk about it. In Glyncorrwg we have been searching actively for alcohol problems for the past 5 years, and about 14% of the men aged 20 or over either have such a problem now, or had one in the past. Many of these have been detected because of high blood pressure apparently resistant to antihypertensive medication. Contrary to most medical and nursing folklore, results of treatment (mainly educational) have been generally good.

The Health Education Council has published leaflets on drinking which are easy to read and understand. The best two we have found are *What's Yours?* and *Will You Need a Stiff Drink After Reading This?*

Sodium and fat in food

Eating the average British diet, men take in about 150mmol, and women about 130mmol of sodium a day. Unfortunately there is no good controlled evidence that moderate reductions of dietary sodium, for example to 100mmol daily or less, have any effect on moderately raised blood pressure in the diastolic range 90–105mmHg. Reductions to about 80mmol or less probably do reduce blood pressure by 5–10mmHg, in people whose pre-treatment pressures are above this threshold, but not enough to make medication unnecessary. As we have explained in Chapter 5, in our experience, even this so-called moderate restriction is difficult for most people to maintain, and our view is that in general these difficulties outweigh the benefits. However, there are individual patients with very high sodium intakes who may benefit from a substantial reduction, and patients with poorly controlled blood pressure who are treated with ACE inhibitors (captopril and enalapril) should reduce sodium intake below 100mmol daily for men and 80mmol daily for women. These and other patients who want to try a low-sodium diet should be helped to do so by giving them the information suggested in Chapter 20, page 218. However, if they find it difficult, and if blood pressure control is not much improved, be ready to permit a return to a normal diet; the evidence of benefit is really very small.

Evidence that a low-fat, high fibre diet reduces blood pressure is much more convincing, and has the added advantage that reduction in animal fats will reduce blood cholesterol. All patients with high blood pressure of any grade should be advised to avoid fried foods, to use semi-skimmed milk, avoid cream, reduce butter, use polyunsaturated margarines and cooking oils, reduce meat, and increase fish, vegetables, fruit and cereals. Recent evidence of benefit from eating more fish is particularly convincing. Time should be made available to discuss this with both patient and spouse, reinforced by the suggested information in Chapter 20, page 218.

FOLLOW-UP OF PATIENTS NOT ON MEDICATION

Follow-up of high blood pressure treated without medication needs to be organised in essentially the same way as the follow-up of patients on antihypertensive drugs. In many cases blood pressure rises and must eventually be treated by drugs, and because all non-drug treatments involve difficult changes in behaviour, fairly frequent follow-up is essential to reinforce education and give patients feedback on their achievement. People who are giving up smoking or trying to lose weight need to be seen at least once a fortnight during the first 6 months, and should never be followed up less than once a year.

ANTIHYPERTENSIVE MEDICATION

For some patients, usually with a mean pre-treatment pressure at or over about 175/105mmHg, control of high blood pressure can be achieved only by drugs. These need regular follow-up both to assess how well the drugs are working and to monitor the effect of treatment on the quality of their lives. In Glyncorrwg we aim to see all of them at least once every three months, more often if their pressure is not controlled to about 160/90mmHg.

Patients who have to take drugs to control their blood pressure will benefit just as much as those who don't from controlling smoking, weight, and cholesterol. Make sure that despite medication, they are helped to become active partners in their care, not just consumers of repeat prescriptions.

Compliance

Compliance means sticking to the rules. Rules are necessary for both care-givers and care-receivers. You will find that if your team has a systematic though intelligently flexible approach, with clearly defined ground rules observed by all staff, patients will generally respond by trying to stick to the rules you give them.

Compliance by patients can be measured in two ways: by measuring *attendance*, calculating the proportion of non-attenders or permanent drop-outs from your clinic, or the proportion of hypertensives seen within a maximum span of (say) 4 months; and by measuring *medication*, counting the number of pills left over at clinic attendances, or observing the dates on which repeat prescriptions are collected; 80% compliance on either of these variables is good; if you get less than 70% you should look critically at your organisation.

Non-attenders and drop-outs

Patients may default from attendance because they can't remember an appointment 3 months ahead; because they work systematic overtime and are afraid of losing their jobs if they take time off; because they are afraid of doctors; because they have to wait a long time at the clinic and then wait again for the chemist to complete their prescription; because they never seem to see the same person at the clinic and don't form any relationship; or because they have not been convinced that they really need treatment.

There are 6 secrets (Ccrets) of success:

Credulity
Continuity
Concern
Comprehension
Contract
and
eConomy.

CREDULITY

Doctors who think they know who will or will not be 'a good patient' are wrong; apart from extremes of age, no sociodemographic variables are consistently associated with either compliance or non-compliance, and both doctors and nurses are poor predictors of patient behaviour. So the first condition for success is an open mind; all patients who really need antihypertensive treatment, from archbishops to alcoholics, should be offered it.

CONTINUITY AND CONCERN

If we want patients to show effective concern for their health, we have got to show effective concern ourselves, by ensuring both continuity of care and a flow rate that allows time to listen and explain. This is where general practice can be so much better than hospital outpatient care, but only with organised and sustained effort.

Continuity is rarely a problem with GPs or practice-employed nurses, but health authority nursing officers in charge of attached nurses do not always understand the need either for continuity, training, or job flexibility. If the nurse in charge of your clinic is changed every couple of months you will never build up an efficient or friendly control programme.

Patients who default clinics twice in succession should be contacted personally, by telephone if they have one or by a home visit. Contact should be made by a nurse rather than a doctor because nurses are more likely to be told the real reasons for default. Whoever does this should try to see the spouse, who may sort everything out for you. If you only have one clinic, it should be held in the evening. Patients should have written appointments asking them to ring your centre if they can't make it. Patients who are afraid to come may still be assiduous in taking their pills; some informal solution can nearly always be found, as long as you accept that half a loaf is better than no bread. A surprisingly common reason for these fears is illiteracy; look for this gently, it can be a minefield.

COMPREHENSION

There are many reasons why patients don't take pills prescribed for them. They may forget; it may not be convenient; the pills may have real or imagined side-effects; there may be too many different pills to take at too many different times each day; they may not believe they need pills because they have no symptoms; or because each time they come for follow-up everything seems OK and they don't understand that treatment is usually a life sentence.

Explaining the nature of hypertension as a permanent rather than episodic condition is the first step to helping patients to understand why they need to take their drugs regularly; the second is to explain and anticipate the side-effects the drugs may have.

CONTRACT

During the first two or three consultations you will get to know the patient both in terms of a personal risk profile, and as a personality with both possibilities and limitations. By the time you know enough about both these aspects to make a realistic treatment plan, this can be negotiated with the patient as a contract. If patients know from the beginning what they are taking on, they are more likely to stick to the rules. If later on they want to change the rules (for example, to take fewer tablets) they are more likely to ask about this openly, knowing that you will listen to their ideas. This is one of several reasons why you should always introduce new drugs one at a time, so that patients can evaluate side-effects and preferences for themselves.

ECONOMY

The more different pills patients must take, and the more often they must remember to take them, the worse their compliance will be. It is partly a matter of having too many things to remember, but even more important is their gut-feeling (or gut-wisdom?) that the more different drugs they take, the higher the risk of side-effects or harmful drug interactions. Don't forget that many of these patients have to take other medications for other conditions, as well as their blood pressure tablets.

Most antihypertensive drugs can now be given in once-daily dosage, and all can be given in twice-daily dosage. Many useful fixed combinations are available, and should be used to assist compliance.

Blood pressures which cannot be controlled

Even in the best hands, about 15–20% of clinic attenders are usually found to have blood pressures seriously out of control (diastolic pressure >100).

The commonest cause of poor control is that patients are not actually taking their tablets, usually for one of the reasons we have just discussed. Whenever you measure blood pressure in a patient on antihypertensive drugs, remember to ask if the tablets have all been taken that day. Omissions just on this particular day are easier to admit, and lead naturally to further sympathetic questions: 'Do you often find it difficult to remember your tablets?', 'Do you think any of these tablets might be upsetting you?' Always ask patients to bring their pills with them, not only for identification but also to estimate numbers left over, assuming that you normally prescribe a bit more than the patient needs from one appointment to the next. A formal tablet count is time-consuming and makes it difficult to avoid a damaging confrontation. A feeling that they're being told off for not complying with treatment may mean dropping out altogether. If patients feel you're prepared to help with suggestions or changes in drugs, you are more likely to hear the true story.

The second commonest reason for poor control is probably alcohol. This can happen in two ways, often both at the same time. Patients who want to drink may imagine that they cannot take any medication at the same time, so they miss out their tablets whenever they go out for a drink; and alcohol taken regularly at a rate of 4 pints of beer a day or more (or the equivalent in wine or spirits) is itself a potent cause of raised blood pressure. Useful clues are raised MCV, GGT, or triglyceride, but the most important investigation is simply to ask patients how much they normally drink each week, going through a typical week one day at a time.

Finally, there seem to be some obese hypertensives whose blood pressures are impossible to control until they lose weight.

REFERENCE

1 Patel C, Marmot MG, Terry DJ. Controlled trial of biofeedback-aided behavioural methods in reducing mild hypertension. *British Medical Journal* 1981; **282:** 2005.

Chapter 14
ANTIHYPERTENSIVE DRUGS

Most readers will either have, or be considering, a regular hypertension clinic run wholly or partly by a nurse. Antihypertensive drugs will be started by doctors, but they may then delegate decisions to raise or reduce dosage to a nurse. There is good evidence from some large hospital clinics in the USA that results are just as good, and errors less common, where nurses follow a standard protocol in starting medication, as well as monitoring progress and modifying dosage. After a year or two of running a clinic, you may well decide to transfer more responsibility to a nurse.

Even nurses who have no responsibility for initiating or modifying treatment must know your criteria for referring the patient to a doctor, and particularly they must be aware of common side-effects from medication, and be able to answer the often surprisingly sophisticated questions patients have about their antihypertensive drugs. Many patients are more likely to talk about their medication worries to a nurse than a doctor.

CHOOSING AND CHANGING ANTIHYPERTENSIVE DRUGS

The *British National Formulary* (BNF) is available in every practice, and is a reliable source of simple information about antihypertensive drugs for nurses as well as doctors.

Within the main groups of antihypertensive drugs, it is important to agree within your team on one or at most two individual drugs, and stick to them so that what must at best be a confused situation, does not become totally incomprehensible. Try also to agree on generic prescribing, generic recording, and generic discussion. There are already 50 different generic drugs listed in the BNF approved for use as antihypertensive agents; it is hardly possible to think at all about what you are doing if you add another 150 brand names.

Five rules for starting, stopping and changing

- Start and stop slowly.
- Make all decisions on more than one reading.
- Don't add new drugs unless you really have to.
- Change one drug at a time.
- Remember that the usual reason for a poor response to treatment is that the tablets are not being taken.

STARTING AND STOPPING

Nearly all side-effects are dose-dependent. Unless you start with the smallest possible dose, you will not find the fortunate minority of patients who respond exceptionally easily, and may saddle them with a lifetime of unnecessary risk. Always *start slowly*, and add increments at weekly or monthly intervals until you either have control, or are forced to add another antihypertensive drug.

Methyldopa, beta-blockers, and clonidine can all cause severe rebound hypertension or angina if they are stopped abruptly. All should be stopped decrementally over 2 or 3 days. Except for diuretics which are only given in low dosage anyway, it seems wise to apply this rule to all antihypertensive medication, and *stop slowly*.

Take a few patient records and look at the points where decisions have been taken to change doses. You will probably find a simple and more or less universal formula:

one deviant measurement → one treatment decision

This is excusable during the initial search for the right dose of a drug, but once control has apparently been achieved, it can't be right. Blood pressure readings are too variable for it to be possible to make intelligent decisions on single readings. If you suddenly get a high reading, don't immediately raise the dose or add another drug; think about possible causes (missed tablets, rushing to the surgery, a full bladder, a very cold day) and *get one or two more readings* over the next day or two, before changing treatment.

Few patients need more than two antihypertensive drugs. When you find yourself thinking about a third drug (which may be the fifth, sixth, or seventh in a patient with other long-term problems such as chronic airways obstruction, arthritis, duodenal ulcer or diabetes) check through other possible causes of failure: non-steroidal anti-inflammatory drugs (NSAIDs) such as indomethacin; unchallenged obesity; heavy alcohol intake; or systematic non-compliance with treatment already prescribed.

Non-compliance is by far the biggest problem with medication. All patients miss tablets some of the time, some patients miss tablets all of the time. Make it a rule that *patients bring all their medication (including treatment for other conditions) with them* at every visit to the clinic, so that both of you know exactly which tablets you are talking about. Patients need encouragement to express their own ideas and fears about their medication, if you are to make an effective contract.

STEPPING DOWN

In patients whose blood pressure has been well controlled, it is worth considering systematic reductions in dosage, and in the number of antihypertensive drugs used; what Finnerty[1] calls step-down therapy. He studied 51 patients whose diastolic pressures had been kept below 90 for 6 months or more, whose blood pressures were measured every 6 weeks. 20 were originally on 3 different antihypertensive drugs, and the other 31 were on 2.

His first step-down was to reduce dosage of 1 drug, and if diastolic pressure remained below 90 for another 6 months, he proceeded to his second step-down, elimination of 1 antihypertensive drug entirely. After 1 year, 13 of the 51 patients had a rise in pressure and had to resume higher medication, but 43 continued to have good control with lower dosage, and 27 were controlled with 1 drug less than before, and this pattern was unchanged during a further 6 months of follow-up. Before the step-down programme, all the patients complained of at least one side-effect of treatment, with a total of 161 complaints; after the programme was completed, 18% of patients reported no change, 26% reported decreased side-effects, and 56% said they were now completely free from side-effects. No patients reported an increase in side-effects.

STEPPING OFF

Though in general patients who have begun treatment on good evidence will need medication for life, and must be educated to accept this from the start without any equivocation, there are exceptions. If good blood pressure control is maintained on lower and lower step-down dosage, there must come a point where you wonder whether antihypertensive drugs are needed at all. As we know only some of the causes of high blood pressure, it is surely possible that there are some patients who have high blood pressure for a few years, but then stop having it. It is even possible that some of these 'cures' are brought about by treatment: that is, without treatment their high blood pressure would have continued to rise, but with careful treatment, some causal cycle is interrupted for long enough for normal blood pressure to be restored, which no longer requires control by medication.

We have found several cases like this in Glyncorrwg, whose original high pressures were well documented, were treated and well controlled for 5 years or more, and who are now being followed up without medication, but still with normal blood pressures. One of them originally had a diastolic pressure of 130mmHg. They are all men, and nearly all were under 40 when they began treatment.

The procedure we followed in Glyncorrwg was first to substitute a placebo tablet for 3 months, with monthly recording of pressure. If blood pressure rose above 150/90 during that time, we could then resume active treatment without a break in continuity; the medication habit is difficult to acquire, and not to be lightly discarded. If blood pressure remained normal, we discussed the position fully with the patient, emphasising the experimental nature and uncertain outcome of the whole procedure, and the need for permanently continued follow-up; every 3 months for the first year, annually thereafter.

These cases are exceptional, but not so rare that you will not eventually find some of them. There seems to be virtually no literature on the subject.

SIDE-EFFECTS

The following side-effects are common with some or all antihypertensive drugs:

- **Tiredness, weakness, depression, and a general feeling of ill-health**. These are particularly common with drugs acting on the brainstem such as methyldopa, reserpine, clonidine, and some of the beta-blockers. They occur occasionally with all antihypertensive drugs, even diuretics and ACE inhibitors, and should always be taken seriously.

- **Glycosuria and gout** are notorious side-effects of thiazide diuretics, often starting after 2 or 3 years of treatment.

- **Faint spells** are common with most antihypertensive drugs, particularly in old people, especially with prazosin. Lying and standing pressures should be measured in these patients.

- **Impotence** is a common side-effect of thiazide diuretics, affecting about 1 man in 5. It is an occasional side-effect of almost all other antihypertensive drugs, and should be asked about specifically about 2 months after starting treatment. If nobody asks, patients are often afraid to discuss the matter, and often attribute it to an effect of hypertension itself rather than the treatment.

- **Wheezing and breathlessness** may be induced by beta-blockers in many people with latent asthma. Beta-blockers (including the cardioselective ones) should never be used in known asthmatics, in whom they can be dangerous. A past history of asthma, often in childhood, is easily overlooked. It is wise always to measure and record PEFR before starting treatment with a beta-blocker, so that any fall in PEFR later on can be recognised.

- **Joint pains** resembling rheumatoid arthritis (SLE syndrome) are common with hydralazine.

- **Diarrhoea, constipation, or nasal stuffiness** are common with many antihypertensive drugs. Whenever any patient on antihypertensive medication reports *any new symptom*, think of the possibility of drug-induced side-effects.

DRUG AND DISEASE INTERACTIONS

Antihypertensive treatment on a mass scale is directed mainly at people in middle and old age, liable to many other ailments which also need treatment. Patients are aware of the possibilities of drug interactions, and unless you discuss these with them, may choose between different medications themselves for fear of precipitating chemical quarrels in their insides, or construct impossibly complex treatment timetables to avoid encounters between rival pills.

The most frequent fear of patients is of interaction between drugs and alcohol. Unfortunately this often leads to omission of medication rather than abstinence. Patients should be warned that the sedative effect of methyldopa may be increased by alcohol, but that alcohol in moderation is not incompatible with other antihypertensive drugs.

Diuretics are often misunderstood. Patients are usually told they are 'water tablets'; this can be a great help when trying to sort out a row of small unlabelled bottles containing various sizes of white tablet, but it is important to explain to patients that though they do indeed promote the outflow of water, they have been prescribed to control blood pressure, not to increase urine output. If they don't understand this, patients may decide that since urine flow is all too free (particularly at night), there is no need to continue the tablets.

The most important and most frequently overlooked interaction is between antihypertensives and NSAIDs such as indomethacin and ibuprofen. Indomethacin increases blood pressure by about 19/9mmHg in patients on diuretics or beta-blockers, almost completely eliminating their hypotensive effect. It is pointless to use NSAIDs for painful but non-inflammatory joint conditions like degenerative arthritis and backache other than ankylosing spondylitis, so part of the answer is to use these drugs only when they are truly necessary. Now that many of them are available in chemists without prescription, it is important to ask patients if they are taking them for headaches, arthritis, or general aches and pains.

There are no important interactions between any commonly used antihypertensive drugs, and drugs used for control of epilepsy or asthma.

COSTS

Sooner or later, primary care teams are likely to become local budget-holders in the National Health Service, so that savings on prescribed drugs might, for example, be available to pay someone to talk to patients about how they actually use their drugs, or help them lose weight, stop smoking, or reduce their blood cholesterol. Even today, economic practice is usually better clinical medicine.

A patient whose blood pressure can be controlled with a diuretic alone (and there are many such people, especially among the elderly), taking bendrofluazide 2.5mg twice a day, costs the nation £2.64 a year (1987 costing). Once daily treatment with chlorthalidone would raise this to £10.32 a year (1987 costing).

If a second drug is required, you might add reserpine, which as 1 combined tablet twice a day would cost only £3.91 (1987 costing) a year. If you were worried about cholesterol levels, you might choose instead prazosin 0.5mg twice a day, which together with bendrofluazide would raise the cost to £30.00 a year. Or you might add atenolol 100mg to chlorthalidone once a day, at a cost of £97.56. Fearing poor compliance, you might prescribe the same beta-blocker combined with chlorthalidone, only raising the cost to £98.04 a year.

Finally, you might decide that the only way to control your patient's blood pressure was an ACE inhibitor, and prescribe enalapril 20mg a day at an annual cost of £157.20 at 1986 prices. If it really were the only way to control pressure this would be justifiable, but for 33 of those you could pay the wages of a full-time member of staff at a higher clerical grade.

REFERENCE

1 Finnerty FA. Step-down therapy in hypertension. *Journal of the American Medical Association* 1981; **246:** 2593.

Chapter 15
FINDING AND CONTROLLING OBESITY

This chapter should be read in conjuction with Chapter 6. If there is anything here which you don't understand, try going back to that chapter.

FINDING OVERWEIGHT PATIENTS

Weight control is an emotive and frustrating business. Most concern about being overweight is shown by women and arises from a conviction that they should look like the advertised image of the desirable woman. Men, however, are at higher risk from obesity (because of their greater liability to coronary disease), and do at least as well as women if they embark on a weight-control programme.

Our concern with obesity is not cosmetic. It is linked with high blood pressure, high blood cholesterol, and diabetes, because weight control favourably affects all three of these conditions.

Overweight can be expressed as *body mass index* (BMI) (see Chapter 6). 'Why bother?' you may ask; obesity is a simple diagnosis with the patient sitting in front of you, and the measurement of height needed for BMI seems superfluous.

There are two reasons for calculating BMI. First, patients want to know their desirable weight, so they can have a personal target. If you know their metric height and weight, desirable weight is BMI 20–25, and life is likely to be shortened over BMI

30. If you have measured metric height, all you have to do is square it, then multiply the product by 25 for desirable weight, or by 30 for maximum safe weight.

Checking a random sample of notes drawn from your shelves may reveal that few patients have been weighed and even fewer measured. As with other screening procedures, you can either take the opportunity to weigh and measure patients as they attend with other complaints, or organise a systematic screening programme for everyone between 20 and 65 years.

To do either of these you will need well-ordered records, an age-sex register, and somewhere in the notes to record your findings. Go back to Chapter 10 if you need help in reorganising your record system.

One reason why it is useful to measure obesity is that it helps to make patients aware, in an objective rather than an emotional way, that they have a weight problem. It is therefore both sensible and important to use the opportunity, while demonstrating BMI, to begin to talk with the patient about eating and diet. As this will take time, a case-finding approach to weight and height measurement may not be appropriate, unless you have long consultation times or patients are likely to return for counselling. You know your own practice organisation and patients; we give only general guidelines for dealing with obese patients which you should adapt to meet your needs, but we think most practices will have to separate the organisation of initial measurements from the organisation of initial counselling.

Do you have balance-arm scales? These are much more expensive than bathroom scales, and heavy to move about. Unlike bathroom scales, which often vary by a pound or two up or down according to temperature and humidity, they *are* accurate. This can be important when you get into arguments with patients who swear they eat nothing but still gain weight. Have you a good height measure? A tape glued to the wall will do, but the neatest gadget, costing only a few pounds, is a sort of reversed steel tape-measure which can be screwed to the door post and pulled down to the top of the patient's head. Don't forget to agree on some standard practice about taking off clothes and shoes, so that whatever you do, it's the same every time. For height measurement, measure the shoe-heel height with the knuckle of your thumb, and subtract it.

HOW WE DO IT

Each practice must tackle ascertainment of obesity in its own way. The procedure described below is the one used in Glyncorrwg. It is imperfect and is not offered as a model, but discussion of real experience may help others to make a start.

We began systematic weighing when we first set up a hypertension clinic in the early 1970s. Weight was one of the measures we applied to hypertensives every time they came to the clinic, usually at intervals of 3 months (the others were blood pressure, smoking, and heart rate). We soon added height, which needs to be recorded only once, so that we could calculate BMI. Those with BMI 30+ were given a red-and-white check label on the spine of their A4 folder, and an 'obesity' entry and BMI value on their summary sheet.

For a long time we did very little about the obesity we found, but because of this system, when we finally developed some enthusiasm for weight control, the figures were there and we could identify our target population. The first effect was unexpected; we found that having an accurate and fairly recent record of weight was helpful in all sorts of other ways in caring for middle-aged patients. Again and again we found it useful to know accurately whether someone had lost or gained weight, in sorting out other causes of illness. So in the end we decided to measure height in everyone aged 20–65, and to aim at weighing everyone at least once every 5 years. It took us about 5 years to get over 90% of them, and we have stayed around that level ever since.

Who should do the weighing and measuring? Whoever has the time and the equipment. If you have a practice nurse in a well-equipped treatment room with accurate scales and height measure, she can see people as they come in, but the work could be done by anyone of the team who has the time. Or weighing could be done by the patient in the waiting room, or perhaps in some quiet place where obese people can weigh themselves without embarrassment; at rather high cost, balance-arm scales are now available which give a digital readout and cannot be misunderstood. It is unwise simply to ask people how tall they are: men particularly tend to add an inch, which makes a big difference to BMI.

If all the practitioners (nurse and medical) have accurate scales and height measures in their rooms, they can also make these measurements during consultations. Where you put the information is as important as getting it, so don't forget to get agreement on where height and weight are to be entered in the records.

Get scales and a vertical ruler

Weigh and measure 'while you wait'

Organise a search

Record it!

Controlling obesity

Eating is an emotionally-charged activity from the moment we find the breast. It can represent communication and warmth as families and friends eat together, or be a compensation for loneliness and depression. Some people just eat compulsively. Advertisers who make it their business to know our weak spots can sell us cream cakes by advising us to spoil ourselves, chocolate bars to treat ourselves and packets of soup to make us warm and an apparently happy family.

For many people losing weight can be an experience which highlights other unsatisfactory parts of their lives. Never underestimate the support your weight-loser will need. One of the reasons why group slimming is usually more successful than individual slimming is that it offers sympathetic support from fellow slimmers, which makes it possible to accept food deprivation.

WHY BOTHER?

Because changing one's diet can be difficult, as well as tough on emotions, helping your patients to find a compelling motive for change is a vital first step to successful weight loss. Not everyone knows the links between high blood pressure, diabetes, arterial disease and obesity, so make sure you tell them in a way they will understand.

For younger patients, the thought of premature death is not always alarming, so you can suggest other good reasons. Most overweight people are conscious of the extra weight they carry, sometimes because they get breathless easily or feel slowed up, and often because of their appearance; listen to what they have to say and feed back to them their reasons for losing weight. There will be many excuses:

> All our family are big,
>
> I've tried before and I can only lose X, then I can't lose any more,
>
> I eat like a bird.

These are probably the most commonly encountered. As with all patient education it is important to discover existing health beliefs before trying to change attitudes. The people who point to obesity in other members of their family are right; the tendency to store excess energy intake as body fat is strongly inherited, and this is why some people eat almost whatever they like without getting fat, while others gain weight at the slightest transgression. The unfairness of this arrangement is the main grievance and excuse for doing nothing about obesity of most overweight people. It's important to explain this to them, and to sympathise with them over the unfairness of evolution in making this arrangement, but in the end you have to insist that there is still only one way for them to lose weight: to ensure that energy intake is less than energy output for as long as it takes to achieve target weight, and then to keep in energy balance for the rest of their lives.

Beliefs about food and dieting will probably astonish you

much of the time, and depress you for the rest. One patient we know believed that eating a pound of grapes each evening would make her thin, and another that he should have one of those meal substitute drinks *added* to each meal. What seems simple and logical to us is a confusing labyrinth to many.

To convince your patients they should bother to lose weight, you will have to find out why they don't, what has happened to previous attempts, what they think will make them thin, correct their inaccuracies and counter their excuses. This investment of time will pay a dividend in well-motivated patients, who understand what they're doing and can maintain a slow but steady weight loss.

SLOW BUT SURE

What most patients really want is a diet which, though it may mean drastically changed eating habits for a week or so, loses three stone in the process. There are many seductive, fast, weight removers on the market, from slimming drinks to cubes unfortunately-named fudge, but you are more likely to help your patients achieve a significant and lasting weight loss if you divert them from the specialist slimming shelves to their own supermarket and butcher, and teach them how to modify their diet less radically but more permanently. Garrow[1] points out that the optimum rate of weight loss is 2kg (4.4lb) a week for the first 4 weeks and 1kg (2.2lb) a week thereafter. Faster decreases are usually the result of starvation which causes loss of fat and lean tissues equally. A slow but steady fall means that only fat is being lost. It is also less likely to be regained because patients who can sustain this slow, steady fall have usually made a permanent and substantial change in eating habits.

Motivation has not only to be high at the start of the diet, but sustained for life. When you plan weight reduction with your patients it means a commitment on your part as well as theirs to regular follow-up over several years.

Some general guidelines follow, to help with individual diet counselling as well as discussion of some other methods of slimming. To fill in the details you will need to familiarise yourself with current research on diet and health: there's a reading list at the end of the chapter, but watch also the popular and medical press to keep up to date.

WHAT DO YOU EAT AND WHEN DO YOU EAT IT?

Most people have an inaccurate idea of how much they eat. Somehow broken biscuits, left-overs from the children's plates, sweets eaten while doing something else are all easily forgotten in the calculation of food intake. One of the easiest ways of bringing this to your would-be dieters' attention is to get them to keep a diary. Explain this as a way of seeing where changes can be made. Emphasise the need for total honesty: if your patients feel their diaries are going to be given marks then they are less likely to be truthful.

As well as knowing exactly what's eaten it is important to know what else is going on during the meal or snack. Were there other people present? Was there an accompanying activity, like reading or watching television? It helps, too, to know how the patient felt when eating; depressed, elated, bored or anxious. As we discussed earlier, many people eat in response to emotions, and it can be helpful for both of you to identify these situations. A recent Health Education Council booklet called *Food for Thought* discusses and illustrates the use of a diet diary. It's well worth reading and having available for patients. If I (BS) kept a diet diary, it would often read thus:

07.45 : Orange juice (small glass)
1 Shredded Wheat, milk, no sugar
Coffee with milk
Read paper, had radio on, in a hurry.

09.30 : Cup coffee with milk while in clinic.

11.00 : Cup coffee with milk, chatted to receptionists; 1 biscuit.

12.45 : Vegetable casserole (potatoes, tomatoes, beans, peas, carrots and cheese)
Baked custard; glass water; talking to colleagues.

13.45 : Cup of coffee with milk while writing at desk.

16.00 : Cup of tea with milk while preparing for evening clinic.

18.00 : Felt very tired so had cup of coffee to revive me for last few patients. Would have eaten but nothing available.

20.00 : Cheese, biscuits, glass wine while watching television.

21.00 : Bored, so had packet crisps and an orange.

22.00 : Decided to treat myself to some chocolate because had had a busy day.

23.00 : Bed with cup herbal tea, no milk. Tired.

There are several areas of my eating patterns which warrant change: I'm always doing something else while I eat, for example reading, talking or watching TV. I seem to snack when I'm bored or tired, and think of food as a treat. I also drink rather a lot of coffee, though I have a reasonably balanced diet.

Why not try keeping one yourself?

MAKING CHANGES

What are you aiming for with your diet counselling? We suggest you consider the following aims:

1 To lower energy intake by encouraging less fat and sugar consumption and more fibre.

2 To raise energy output by encouraging exercise.

3 To bring BMI down to 25 or 30 and keep it there. This is the patient's target, not yours, and he or she must genuinely accept it as reasonable.

Base the changes you suggest on your patient's diary.

The Health Education Council's booklets *Look After Yourself, Beating Heart Disease* and *Food for Thought* all have good suggestions about increasing fibre, decreasing fat and sugar and eating well-balanced meals.

Read these yourself, as well as a reliable book on nutrition (see p. 173). Learn to identify the main sources of fat in your patients' diets.

Make changes gradually, and ensure that they are practical; how will your suggestion affect the meal preparation for a family, for example? Eventually both you and your patients will have to face the need to cut down food so that energy intake is less than output. This is the hardest part of weight loss, but can be made easier by giving up 'empty calories', like alcohol, sweet fizzy drinks, and other quickly burned sugars. Again, use the patient's diet diary to discover where energy intake can be trimmed most easily.

KEEP MOVING

An exercise programme undertaken at the same time as diet changes makes weight loss easier. Little of this is from the direct effect of extra energy expenditure (unless you become a 4-minute miler); most of the benefit of exercise seems to come from changed attitudes to life in general, including eating, smoking, and a greater enjoyment of life and therefore higher motivation to maintain health. There may also be a small increase in metabolic rate. Regular exercise seems to make people generally more health conscious and thus to reduce appetite. It also helps to prevent coronary heart disease by lowering blood low-density (LDL) and raising high-density (HDL) cholesterol, and by lowering blood pressure. Lung and heart functions improve, so that even patients who do get heart attacks are more likely to survive them. There is also some evidence in diabetics that energy throughput is important, not just energy balance; diabetics who both consume and use very little energy do less well than those who take in a lot of energy but use it up vigorously in a physically active life.

Patients can build up an exercise schedule by starting with

half-an-hour's brisk walking each day, gradually moving to an appropriate sport or activity. Exercises like weight-lifting and press-ups, which rely on short, sharp bursts of energy, use a chemical system in muscle cells which does not need oxygen; this is called *anaerobic exercise*. It can cause steep though transient rises in blood pressure which can be dangerous. Endurance exercises, such as jogging, walking or swimming, use a different chemical system in the same muscle cells, which depends on oxygen, and this *aerobic exercise* seems to be a much better way to become and to stay fit. The circulatory system responds to regular endurance exercise by increasing the strength and efficiency of heartbeats, by improving the circulation of blood within the heart muscle itself, and probably by removing some of the cholesterol deposited in the artery walls, particularly in the coronary arteries, which impede the circulation of blood.

The Health Education Council booklets *Look After Yourself* and *Looking After Yourself* give sound schedules for building up exercise routines. You could also usefully read the sensible *Sunday Times Body Book*, as well as having it available for patients to borrow. It gives sound advice about diet and exercise. Like diet, exercise routines take a while to build up and must be maintained over a long period to have beneficial effects. Regular exercise is important: 4 sessions of 20 minutes each in a week seems to be the minimum time for any real improvement in fitness.

Remember to take joint pain into account in exercise counselling. Swimming is particularly helpful in these cases, and for obese or elderly people generally, because the submerged body is almost weightless, and movements which are impossible out of the water can be easily performed in it. Other advantages of swimming are that it is usually an individually performed activity, so that people can move at their own pace, heated indoor swimming baths are available in most communities and can be used in all weathers, and adult learning classes are usually available, with instructors who can teach people who have never learned to swim.

Another possibility for many people is cycling. Stationary exercise bikes are available for people who are unwilling or unable to use a real bike for work or leisure, at prices varying from about £60–£300, depending on their strength and sophistication. Those offered cheaper than this are too flimsy to be worth buying. Real cycling is much better for most people, and is more likely to become a regular exercise commitment. Can a bike be used for all or part of the daily journey to and from work? Good machines are available from about £70 new, much less secondhand.

For both cycling and jogging, consider the safety of your practice area for lone joggers and cyclists. You may need to make representations to your county council for improvement of cycle paths, or to your borough council for improved footpaths, playing fields, or times of access to swimming pools. Half a day spent on local research could yield not only useful information but friendly contacts too.

MAKING TIME FOR INDIVIDUAL AND GROUP COUNSELLING

Major lifestyle changes, particularly those relating to eating, can be difficult to initiate and impossible to maintain without help. The type of help patients need depends on their preference for group or individual counselling.

What help can you offer in your practice? Remember that for each patient, individual teaching will take perhaps 20 minutes initially, and follow-up support may take another 10 minutes every 2–4 weeks, for perhaps 12–18 months. Has anyone the time to do that in your practice? The immediate answer is almost certainly 'no', but you may find a solution by delegating part or all of your individual counselling to a new person squeezed somehow into the Red Book definition of reimbursable ancillary staff, or (if you have a progressive and imaginative health authority) seconded from their staff.

INDIVIDUAL DIET COUNSELLING

As we are constantly stressing the importance of relevant health teaching, you will not be surprised that we recommend that all your patients have an initial opportunity for one-to-one teaching and advice on all health risks (not only diet).

Initial sessions will take at least 20 minutes a patient to allow time for you to explain why you are interested in your patients' weight and for them to tell you whether and how they can diet. Follow-up sessions can be shorter, perhaps 5–10 minutes, though you will still need time to discuss difficulties; but here there is the less-time-consuming alternative of group sessions.

So far, personalised advice of this kind has been thought of as the responsibility of doctors but because few NHS practitioners have anything like the amount of time it needs, few have accepted it in any systematic way.

Though moral support and encouragement can probably be given as effectively by an interested and sympathetic nurse, receptionist, or even another successful dieter, this is not the only component of either initial counselling or follow-up. It is important not to underestimate the amount of knowledge required to field the wide variety of intelligent questions patients will fire at you. The information given in Chapter 6 is really a minimum. Without this, there is a temptation to fall back on the mixture of common sense and uncritical contemporary superstition we can all produce off the tops of our heads. Even though all doctors and some nurses have had an education in basic physiology and are therefore assumed to know all these answers, the truth is that most of this is quickly forgotten once they have passed their exams, the only exceptions being those parts of knowledge which are used all the time in their daily work. Because little of this daily work has been preventive, most of us have to relearn the physiology we once knew, and this requires time. All honest, intelligent, literate, and well-motivated people can learn, but they will need specific, relevant, and realistic teaching, and this is not easy to find.

If 12% of your practice population aged 20–64 have BMI at or over 30, how many patients will that involve? In an average practice list of 2200 you are likely to find 1232 (56%) aged 20–64, and 148 of these will have this degree of obesity. At 20 minutes each that represents about 49 counselling hours for initial consultations alone. If all follow-up support is done individually in 5 or 10 minute encounters once a month, this will add another 2–5 hours a week.

GROUP TEACHING AND SUPPORT

Counselling time can be reduced by dealing with people in groups rather than individually. Many people find that the impetus to begin and continue losing weight comes from talking to other people with the same problems. Arranging for all your slimmers to meet once a week, to be weighed and to talk about their difficulties, could provide the support they need and save you time. If your local authority (as in Birmingham and London) employs a community dietician or nutritionist, she might be able to run such a group, or you might persuade your health authority to make a hospital nutritionist or dietician available for a session. Such meetings are also a useful venue for other people with a message to come along and give their views. A physiotherapist from your local hospital, or instructors from local sports and swimming centres, might be persuaded to talk about and teach exercise schedules. If your practice staff have no time to organise and lead a group, could your health visitor or community nurse do so? If none of your staff is able to organise a group within your practice, what about enlisting the help of other existing local groups? Weight Watchers seem to be successful, but they are a strictly commercial organisation and in our experience are not interested in sharing care on a non-profit basis. You may need to check the suitability of their diet for patients with high cholesterol levels. Finally, you may find people in your community willing to run such a group voluntarily.

All such patient groups are easier to set up than to maintain. People with a definite 'disease' label, such as hypertensives and diabetics, may fairly easily accept attendance at groups sessions as a regular and permanent part of their lives. Although weight problems are just as permanent, few weight-losing groups last longer than a year or so. They have a beginning, a middle, and an end, and if you have to rely on voluntary unpaid help, lay or professional, it is essential to recognise this from the start, and plan the end before it occurs spontaneously through loss of interest among participants or exhaustion of those in charge. Paid workers have a huge advantage both in permanence, and in accountability; work given free is difficult to criticise, but without criticism you may eventually run into serious problems with the outsize personalities who tend to volunteer.

A spin-off from organising such a group is motivation for the organiser. Diet counselling, important though it is, is not always exciting, and any boredom will show. Talking to others with interest in and knowledge of the subject revitalises waning enthusiasm.

MANY DISEASES, ONE DIET

The control of obesity, high blood cholesterol, and diabetes, fortunately all call for the same changes in diet:

Energy input reduced below energy output, until target weight is attained, input balanced with output thereafter, by reducing intake of high-energy foods like sugar and fats, and by eating only at mealtimes.

Animal (saturated) fats reduced as far as possible; by eating less meat and then only lean cuts with visible fat removed, by drinking skimmed or semi-skimmed milk and avoiding cream, by reducing butter and cheese, and by avoiding the concealed and usually forgotten fats in biscuits, cakes, and shortbread; by *substituting vegetable (unsaturated) fats*, soft margarines, sunflower oil, and *substituting fish for meat*; and by grilling, steaming, or microwave cooking rather than frying.

Fibre increased by eating more raw or lightly-cooked fruit, vegetables, and unrefined cereals; wholemeal bread, brown rice, and jacket potatoes.

SALT AND SODIUM

People with high blood pressure who add a lot of salt to their food, eat a lot of salty foods like salted nuts, crisps, kippers and strong cheeses, or eat Chinese take-away foods with added monosodium glutamate, should be encouraged to reduce or stop these foods, and should also be warned that most prepared foods (tins and ready-cooked frozen foods) have very large amounts of added salt. However, even for these people, it seems to be more important to reduce fat than to reduce salt, and as most people find it difficult to make both these changes at once, priority should be given to reducing fat and increasing fruit and vegetables. There is still no convincing evidence that people with normal or borderline blood pressures below 150/90 benefit from low salt diets, and you should not make life even more difficult for them by adding this to their other tasks.

REFERENCE

1 Garrow JS. *Treat obesity seriously: a clinical manual*. Edinburgh: Churchill Livingstone, 1981.

FURTHER READING

Basky EJ, Fentam P. *Exercise: the facts*. Oxford: Oxford University Press, 1981.

Gillie O, Raby S. *The Sunday Times body book*. London: Hutchinson, 1984

Hart CR (ed.). *Screening in general practice*. Edinburgh: Churchill Livingstone, 1975.

Chapter 16
FINDING AND CONTROLLING HIGH BLOOD CHOLESTEROL

Of the 3 major risk factors for coronary heart disease (smoking, high blood pressure, and high blood cholesterol), cholesterol is both the most fundamental and the most neglected.

It is the most fundamental in that people with a truly normal blood cholesterol, below 5mmol (200mg)/dl, hardly ever get coronary heart attacks even if they smoke and have high blood pressure, though they do get lung cancer and stroke. Only 10% of adult men in Britain have a blood cholesterol as low as this, and all above this level are at risk for coronary disease. Experts who favour a so-called 'high-risk' policy, want us to concentrate our clinical effort on the top 10–20% of the range of blood cholesterols.[1] Even if this were 100% effective, it would identify only 18–32% of those who will suffer fatal or non-fatal coronary heart attacks during the next 5 years,[2] and its advocates seem not to understand that even this limited objective is far beyond the resources of any hospital outpatient department, because of the enormous numbers involved.

Let us suppose that we concentrate on men aged 40–59 (15% of the whole population), with blood cholesterols in the top 20% of the range. An average general practice with 2000 patients will then include 300 men whose cholesterol must be measured, of whom 60 will have blood cholesterols in the top 20% of the range, needing personal dietary advice and follow-up. It is hardly surprising that even the most innovative practices have generally avoided this painful and presently impracticable conclusion, and preferred to concentrate on blood pressure control, not perhaps because it is more effective, but because numbers appear more manageable, and treatment has involved pills rather than changed behaviour.

The only other alternative is the so-called 'population approach', in which individual measurements are ignored and effort is concentrated on education about healthier eating, directed at the general public. Some experts advocate concentration on children and adolescents (because they might benefit most), others advocate concentration on adults aged 35–54, because being at higher risk, they may be the most likely to act upon advice while there is still time for it to be effective.

Our impression is that none of the experts on either side of this dispute has fully thought out the implications of all this for the organisation of care. The 'high-risk' strategy is on such a mass scale that general practitioners in their present state are unable even to contemplate it (let alone hospital specialists), and in reality it is confined to a few people who find their way into teaching hospital departments, or buy their way into BUPA screening. The 'population approach' is bigger still, so big that most primary care teams don't really feel involved; apart from leaving some leaflets in the waiting room, we have abdicated the educational task to the mass media, and those parts of the food industry which see new opportunities for profit from a more health-conscious public. Either way, those who most need the information are least likely to get it. We can and should find a better way than either of these.

WHOSE BLOOD CHOLESTEROL SHOULD BE MEASURED?

Total blood cholesterol can now be measured reliably, cheaply, and easily on non-fasting, casual samples of clotted blood. It gives less information about risk than a full lipid profile, including HDL cholesterol, but this is a more expensive procedure with a greater laboratory error.

Obviously you will want to measure total cholesterol in anyone with possible angina or claudication. We think you should also measure it at least once in all hypertensives and diabetics (you will be taking blood from these anyway for other purposes, and if you use Vacutainers there is no problem about taking further samples while you are in the vein), and in anyone with a history of coronary heart disease under age 60 in a parent or sibling. You may also find you have more success in counselling smokers if you assess all their other risk factors, including total cholesterol. Finally, people interested enough to ask for their blood cholesterol to be measured deserve to have that information.

Blood cholesterol should also be measured in those women on oral contraceptives who insist on continuing to smoke, to assist in assessing their personal risk from doing so. It is particularly important to measure cholesterol in women diabetics, who are at the same risk of coronary disease as men.

Here is a suggested minimum list:

Hypertensives

Diabetics

People with angina or claudication

Men with a history of coronary disease under 60 in a parent or sibling

Women on the pill who continue to smoke.

WHO SHOULD BE FOLLOWED UP AND HOW?

All hypertensives, diabetics, and people with symptoms of arterial disease need dietary advice and follow-up. In the other groups, initial dietary advice should be given to all, and those with total blood cholesterol at 7.0mmol (270mg)/dl should be followed up.

Dietary advice should follow the pattern given in Chapter 7 and repeated in Chapter 20. Follow-up should include a further measurement of total cholesterol about 3 months after starting a cholesterol-lowering diet, with checks perhaps once a year or every 18 months thereafter. Together with frequent measurement of body weight, these checks are important feedback, helping patients to continue their efforts.

Like the obese, but even more so, people with high blood cholesterol vary in their response to diet, some achieving a reduction of as much as 20% with little difficulty, others as little as 5% or less despite great effort. Those who find it difficult or impossible need reassurance that reduction of high cholesterol is only one way to reduce risk, and should be encouraged to concentrate on others.

REFERENCES

1 Oliver MF. Strategies for preventing and screening for coronary heart disease. *British Heart Journal* 1985;**54**:1.
2 Shaper AG, Pocock SJ. British blood cholesterol values and the American consensus. *British Medical Journal* 1985;**291**:480.

Chapter 17
FINDING AND CONTROLLING DIABETES

Only 1% of diabetics die of diabetic coma, whereas 72% die of coronary heart disease, stroke, or kidney failure, all of which can be prevented or delayed by control of the same three major risk factors as in non-diabetics; smoking, high blood pressure, and high blood cholesterol. To a considerable and usually underestimated extent, good care of diabetics, particularly of maturity-onset, non-insulin-dependent diabetics, consists of conscientious control of these cardiovascular rather than specifically diabetic risks. At 2% of the population, they are the smallest easily-defined group at very high risk of coronary heart disease and stroke, so they are a particularly attractive first target for any practice keen to make a start in improving its anticipatory care.

No undiscovered diabetic should ever get past any reasonable screening programme. Of all detectable but often symptomless conditions, diabetes is one of the cheapest and easiest to identify, and can be one of the most rewarding to manage; and, as we explained in Chapter 6, diabetics gain most from organised prevention and anticipatory care of arterial disease, and suffer most from the lack of an organised programme.

FIRST STEPS

Here are some guidelines and reminders to help you plan your strategies.

As before, the first step is to get the practice team to agree on the importance and feasibility of discovering all diabetics and controlling their disorder accurately. This agreement should not be taken for granted; many GPs (and even some hospital physicians) still believe that only insulin-dependent diabetics run serious risks of premature death, that accurate control of maturity-onset, non-insulin-dependent diabetes does little to reduce such risk as there is, and that maturity-onset diabetics are in any case more or less impervious to advice.

Maturity-onset diabetics themselves tend to underestimate the risks of their condition, and once they have understood that they don't need injections, are pleased to find that they apparently have a minor illness which can be treated casually. So your second obstacle will be the complacency of many patients.

INTENSIVE SCREENING OR EXTENSIVE CASE-FINDING?

As we all know, but occasionally forget, urine should be tested for glucose whenever you see men or women with:

- all forms of arterial disease, coronary heart attacks, angina, claudication, transient brain ischaemia and stroke,
- obesity in middle or old age,
- thirst or getting up at night to pass urine,
- otherwise unexplained weight loss, particularly in those previously overweight,
- recurrent genital candidiasis (thrush),
- recurrent intertrigo,
- recurrent skin sepsis,
- recurrent urine infections,
- recurrent itching,
- leg ulcers and other skin lesions that won't heal,
- cataract,
- impotence,
- a history of diabetes in a parent or sibling,
- a history of very big babies or glycosuria in pregnancy.

Testing casual samples of urine is not enough when you have such positive grounds for suspicion; you should arrange for a sample of urine to be collected about 2 hours after the main meal of the day. Even this may not be sufficient in old people, whose kidneys often have a higher threshold for blood glucose; you can only rule out diabetes in these people by blood tests.

Of course this sort of case-finding is elementary, and on good days none of us ever forgets to test urine. You will find middle-aged obese diabetics, rather than acutely ill patients. If this process is applied systematically to all patients attending over 5 years or so, you won't miss much, though because diabetes increases with age, you will continue to find new cases among people who have already been tested. Of the giant obese (BMI 40+), nearly all eventually develop diabetes, and in all the symptom groups listed, you have to keep on looking, particularly if they continue to gain weight.

Providing you really are applying these search criteria systematically, there is probably little to be gained by organising any formal screening. Insulin-dependent diabetics usually present quickly after onset of their disease, and are rarely picked up by screening.

REDISCOVERING KNOWN DIABETICS

The biggest problem is not finding new diabetics, but giving proper care to those we already know. Or do we? Unless you already keep a register of diabetics, or have some system for flagging their records, there is no way you can check whether or how well they are being looked after by anyone. If there is no register, the best way to find those of your diabetics on medication is to watch out for repeat prescriptions for antidiabetic drugs. You may pick up some of those on diet only by repeat prescriptions for urine-testing tablets and sticks. Even then there will certainly be gaps.

Once you have a list of known diabetics, you can audit their care. Try to work out from the records whether they are attending a hospital clinic, or your own nurses or doctors, or both, or perhaps no one at all. General practice is certainly the best place to follow up maturity-onset diabetes, but only if it is really well organised and the whole team has a thorough knowledge of the requirements for safe monitoring. Until you are sure about this, don't be in too much of a hurry to pull back your patients from the hospital clinic.

Your eventual aim is likely to be some kind of shared care for insulin-dependent diabetics, and primary team care for non-insulin-dependent diabetics, backed up by specialist advice when you need it. If you have agreed to organise diabetic care in your practice, arrange to meet your local diabetologist and the diabetic nurse or dietician; they will probably be helpful in offering advice and perhaps training to members of your team, you may be able to agree on criteria for specialist referral and return to team care, and they may offer a dietary adviser for a clinic if you decide to run one. All hospital diabetic clinics are overworked, and diabetologists are usually grateful for any chance to offload their non-insulin-dependent patients to any practice prepared to accept serious continuing responsibility.

A PRACTICE DIABETIC CLINIC?

In some places diabetic mini-clinics are held in GPs' surgeries, though the patients are sent for through hospital administration and their care is still seen as a hospital extension. This really does make diabetes a speciality, and the danger is that other aspects of patients' health may be ignored. You may feel that having your own clinic set aside only for diabetics could have this effect too, though it's difficult to be sure you are doing all that is necessary for your diabetic patients during routine sessions, and even harder to follow them up regularly.

One option is to hold a special session for diabetic patients at the end or beginning of a routine surgery. In that way, whoever is seeing the patients is geared to the everyday, whole person care required by general or nurse practitioners and the diabetic patients mingle and wait with all-comers. But you lose the considerable advantages of developing the diabetics as a self-educating, mutually supportive group, you may find it difficult to get specialised nursing help for such small numbers and so short a time, and if the numbers are bigger, who will want to see them before or after a busy general session?

About 1% of the population in your practice is likely to be known to have diabetes, rather more than 20 patients in an average practice population of 2100, and about two-thirds of these will be non-insulin dependent. If you undertake intensive case-finding in the way we suggest, known diabetics will increase to about 2% of the population, about 40 patients in an average practice, and nearly all of the new ones will be non-insulin dependent. Most diabetologists agree that people with uncomplicated maturity-onset diabetes rarely need to be seen more than twice a year, providing that when they are seen, a few simple monitoring procedures are conscientiously performed. This means an average initial annual workload of 40 consultations, rising eventually to about 80. You might manage easily with a quarterly clinic to begin with, perhaps later increasing to monthly; the workload is much less than with a blood pressure clinic because the numbers are one-fifth as big, though more monitoring procedures are needed, and the higher proportion of elderly people means that you must work more slowly.

Why have a clinic at all? The case for concentrating diabetic care in a clinic is stronger even for diabetes than for hypertension. It is generally understood that diabetics need to understand the nature of their problem and that diet is a very important part of their care, and diabetic nurses and dieticians already exist who accept this, and are prepared to give it the necessary time and patience (none of this is yet true of hypertension). If you don't run a clinic, you can't get such people to help you. The numbers are more manageable than for hypertension, the risks are higher, and the opportunities for making a real difference to outcome are correspondingly greater. Finally, running your own diabetic clinic will probably give your doctors, nurses, and office staff a continuing and mutually beneficial contact with their opposite numbers in hospital, which is for some reason a much rarer consequence of good hypertension control.

To hold a clinic you will need a doctor and a nurse. A doctor may be able to run a general session concurrently, only seeing problem patients and checking optic fundi, and is likely to need less than a third of the time spent by the nurse. You will need a room to hold it in, with a dark room for examining fundi and preferably with a direct access to a toilet. You will need clerical back-up to organise the clinic and call up the patients, to handle the records during the clinic, and to help you go through the list of non-attenders at the end. Even very junior office staff may be helpful in doing blood and urine tests, lending books, giving out pamphlets, and may eventually learn to help with diet counselling and smoking control.

MONITORING DIABETES

You need a good book on management of diabetes in general practice, and this is not it. We only go into detail regarding prevention of arterial disease in diabetics, but since this is what most of them die of, its importance is hard to exaggerate.

Here is our list of essential tasks:

Every six months

Take blood for glycosylated haemoglobin (HbA1c). This test has transformed the practical management of diabetics by giving us a valid indicator of the average blood glucose level over the previous 3 months. Ideally, it should be less than 9%; if it is over 12%, management needs substantial change. Obviously, there is no point in repeating it in less than 2 or 3 months. If you can, arrange for patients to come a week before the clinic for blood to be taken, so that you have the result when they see you. Spot blood glucose estimations are now easy with BM sticks (which are just as good as an electronic meter), but much less informative than HbA1c.

Look at the patients' urine or blood glucose chart and discuss it.

Ask about any problems, specifically including:

chest pain
bladder troubles
problems with sex function

leg pains and numbness
foot troubles
skin rashes and sores
problems with vision.

Ask if the patient still smokes, and decide whether to tackle the problem again on this occasion.

Ask about alcohol intake: estimate in units (+ pints, glasses, or measures) per week.

Check blood pressure.

Weigh the patient and check against an agreed target.

Look at the patients' medication (not just antidiabetic agents, *all* medication). Always ask patients to bring their pills with them in their original containers.

Ask again about any problems.

Once a year

Check vision of each eye separately through a pinhole, or using the patient's usual near and distance glasses.

Examine both fundi, in a dark place, pupils dilated with a rapid mydriatic.

Test urine for protein.

Check foot and ankle pulses and look at toes.

Check ankle reflexes with the patient kneeling on a chair.

Check blood urea and creatinine.

Check *mean corpuscular volume* (MCV) and *gamma glutamyl*

transferase (GGT) if there are any indications of excessive alcohol intake.

In our experience, it is impossible to remember to do all these things unless they are written out as a checklist, either kept in the notes, or retained by the patient.

Don't lose them!
After you have discovered who are the diabetics in your practice how are you going to keep track of them? As with hypertensives, most people find a card index best.

FRONT

JONES, EDWARD	
21 Any Street	d.o.b. 11.10.32
Hightown	
Tel: 683	
Diabetes diagnosed 1983.	
Family history:	Father diabetic, late onset, died age 63 Mother, alive and well.
Children:	Peter, 1958 Elizabeth, 1961 (Now Barrett)

BACK

Drugs – None; dietary control only

July 1983	–	Review monthly
January 1984	–	Review 2/12
August 1984	–	Review 3/12
November 1984	–	Did not attend – appt. sent
December 1984	–	Review 3/12

An appointment book completes this system, so that you know who hasn't turned up to a clinic and can send for them again. If you aim to see all your diabetics once every 6 months, then defaulters should be picked up by an annual audit, chasing defaulters (within reason) to attend at any time (your clinic times may have been difficult for them). Much of this can be done by telephone, if you are lucky enough to have most of your patients with telephones.

It is useful for diabetics to carry their own card, detailing their current treatment, the date and time of their next visit, with instructions about action to be taken by the patient or family in the event of intercurrent illness, and by bystanders in the event of coma from low blood-glucose.

Diet

'Dietary control should not be considered as failed, if it has never been seriously tried.'

If these words seem familiar, it's because they have been taken from Chapter 6. They refer to dietary control of diabetes, and we repeat them here because they are so important. Patients often have strong and inaccurate health beliefs about diabetes, confusing maturity-onset diabetes with the insulin-dependent variety, either believing the disease to be too serious to control by diet alone, or that if diet alone can control it, it must be trivial. In particular, most patients believe that as sugar in the urine is the hallmark of diabetes, sugar in food must be its principal cause, and that all they have to do is to stop eating sugar. This belief will continue to be held until someone with more authority corrects it.

Are you sure you understand the link between obesity and diabetes yourself? How about the links between diabetes and exercise, or high fibre diets and cholesterol? If not, have another look at Chapters 6 and 7.

All diabetics should be encouraged to become active members of the British Diabetic Association, 10 Queen Anne Street, London W1M 0BD (01–323 1531), which has local branches in most large towns and cities and produces a wide range of educational material.

PROTOCOL FOR NURSE-RUN FOLLOW-UP OF NON-INSULIN-DEPENDENT DIABETICS

This is the protocol we have used at Glyncorrwg for many years; it is only a guide, and should be modified to suit your local requirements.

GPs with good, up-to-date hospital training in the care of insulin-dependent diabetes can manage all but the most complicated insulin-dependent diabetics, but most GPs will probably want to leave insulin-dependent diabetics to hospital clinics, perhaps with some shared management. This protocol refers only to care of maturity-onset, non-insulin-dependent diabetics.

Diabetic clinics can be much less frequent than hypertension clinics, because there are 5 times fewer diabetics than hypertensives in need of drug treatment, and because control of maturity-onset diabetes is generally more stable than control of high blood pressure. In Glyncorrwg we found that the number of patients (30) was too small to justify a separate clinic, and we now follow up our diabetics in the hypertension clinic, adding the specific diabetic data to the routinely collected hypertension data. Because coronary disease and stroke are such big risks for diabetics, many of the procedures are the same for both groups, and our experience has been that half the diabetics need treatment for hypertension anyway. If the doctors in your practice stick to the principle of personal lists, they also may decide to group diabetics and hypertensives together in one clinic. With or without a clinic, with diabetics and hypertensives seen separately or together, routine follow-up can be run by a practice nurse, with a doctor concurrently available for advice and referral.

Ascertainment, initial diagnostic work-up, and initiation of patient education and treatment are all done in ordinary sessions and should be completed before relegation to follow-up. You should normally deal only with people already stabilised on treatment and fairly well controlled.

The *aims* of the clinic are:

1 To review patients' records of their own urine or blood glucose tests, check urine for protein, measure glycosylated haemoglobin (HbA1c), blood pressure, body weight, current smoking, ankle pulses, and ankle reflexes in all maturity-onset diabetics at least once every 6 months, and check blood urea and creatinine once every 5 years.
2 To test acuity of vision using standard test type in each eye

separately (you can do this), and search both optic fundi through dilated pupils for microaneurysms and proliferative arteriolar damage (a doctor must do this), at least once a year.
3 To control glycosylated haemoglobin (HbA1c) below 9% (good control), or 12% (partial control).
4 To control BMI (metric weight divided by the square of metric height) below 26 (good control) or 30 (partial control).
5 To verify that patients understand their diet and medication, and if not, explain it to them.
6 To enquire about significant symptoms of diabetic complications; central chest pain, leg pain or numbness, burning urine, genital itching or rash, deteriorating vision, loss of erection.
7 In patients who still smoke, to enquire about respiratory symptoms, and use these or other opportunities to re-open negotiations on stopping when the time seems right to do this.

Procedures

Whenever a new diabetic patient is detected, the patient's record will be marked with a *brown tab* on the spine, and the name and address will be noted and given to you. Before the next clinic you should enter the name, address, and telephone number if any on a card, which you should place in a *boxed card-index* containing all diabetics known to the practice, grouped in clinic date order so that everyone should be seen not less than once every 6 months. At each clinic each of these cards should be date-stamped, with a note on whether the patient attended or defaulted. No other information should go on this card, except for anything which may help to improve contact. For example, note people who are housebound and will need a visit from the doctor or community nurse, or who have special difficulties such as odd shifts, or can't sit in the waiting room because of phobic symptoms.

One week *before the clinic*, look through the group listed for it and ask the receptionist to extract these patients' records. Look at the last entry. If the patient has had a diabetes check within the last 6 months and was well controlled, give them a new date 6 months ahead, enter this on the card, and put it back in the box at the appropriate date. If the patient seems to be housebound, ask the practice manager to give the visit either to one of the doctors or to a community nurse, whichever was responsible for the last entry. If the patient defaulted the last clinic, consider ringing them up or visiting them at home to find out what their difficulty is in attending. For all the others, send out a written invitation to attend the clinic, with an appointment time.

At the clinic start seeing patients as soon as they begin to arrive, usually 15 minutes or so before the doctor is due to arrive. Enter the date, and if the patient has defaulted or sent an apology, record this. Ask patients how they have been since their last clinic visit, and have a look at the last entry in their records to see if something new has happened since then. Ask each patient to show you his or her tablets (whatever they are prescribed for, not only diabetes), which should *always* be brought to the clinic, and check that they are being taken as recorded on the repeat prescription sheet. Then measure and record the following data:

Blood pressure. Use phase 5 (disappearance of sound) for diastolic pressure, and record to the nearest 2mmHg, with the mercury descending at a rate of roughly 2mm per pulse beat. Tell the patient the result.

Pulse rate. Count pulse over 15sec and multiply by 4.

Current smoking in cigarettes a day.

Weight in kilograms. Target weight is BMI less than 26 (ideal weight) or 30 (maximum safe weight).

Posterior tibial and dorsalis pedis pulses (present or absent), Achilles tendon reflexes (present or absent), and evidence of dermatitis, ulcers, or footrot.

Finally, take venous blood for glycosylated haemoglobin. If you do this at the clinic, you will have to recall the patient if the result is unsatisfactory. A better alternative is to arrange for all patients to attend one week before their appointments just to have the blood taken, so that the result of HbA1c is available for discussion at the clinic. HbA1c is the best single indicator of the quality of control, and ideally should be kept around 8–9%.

Ask all patients if, for *any* reason, they would like to see the doctor. The doctor will be seeing a few other non-diabetic patients, but he or she will be under less pressure than you are and *all* patients who want to see the doctor should do so.

Refer patients to the doctor if:

glycosylated haemoglobin (HbA1c) is over 11%, or most urine tests show positive glycosuria;

you find protein in the urine for the first time, or there is any change in symptoms or signs;

systolic pressure is over 160mmHg or diastolic pressure is over 90mmHg;

you think, and the patient agrees, that it would be useful to tackle smoking again and discussion with the doctor could help in this;

you think, and the patient agrees, that it would be useful to tackle obesity again and discussion with the doctor could help in this;

the patient has not seen a doctor for a year or more;

you are worried for any reason about the patient.

If the doctor is doubtful about the patient's vision or retinal appearance, don't forget that the patient's optician may be able to give a useful opinion.

On average, we usually expect about one-third of the patients to need referral to the doctor.

After the clinic discuss any interesting or difficult cases, and each defaulter, with the doctor. Decide on action to be taken in respect of each defaulter.

ONCE EVERY 6 MONTHS:
Check that every record with a brown tab has a card in the boxed index.
Check every card in the index to see that everyone in it has either been seen, or that arrangements are in hand for them to be seen .

This will take you an hour or two. If you need more time, raise this at the next practice staff meeting.

PART FOUR: DIVISIONS OF LABOUR

Chapter 18
EDUCATION AND TRAINING

OBJECTIVES

The objectives of education may be summarised under three headings.

1 To improve knowledge
2 To improve skills
3 To improve application of skills.

Any training programme, whether designed for yourself or for other people, must aim at *all* of these objectives, for without concentrating specifically on the third, application of skills, there is no guarantee that new knowledge or skills will be put into practice.

Improving knowledge

The traditional approach to education has been to treat the mind as an empty vessel, and pour knowledge in as water is poured from a jug.

This is inaccurate for people are rarely completely ignorant about any topic. Most of us already have a minestrone of knowledge, a jumbled up mixture of assertions, facts, relationships and rules. Some new ingredients are often necessary, but it is usually just as important to syphon off incorrect beliefs as to add new facts. It is also important to stir up the facts people already have and help them put these in better order, for they often have the information they need, but are unable to marshal it appropriately.

Improving knowledge, therefore, consists of three main approaches.

1 Helping people to identify and discard inaccurate, useless or harmful information.
2 Helping them to sort out information they already have.
3 Helping them to acquire the facts they need to complement those they already have.

FACTS AND RULES

People need facts, for example the complicated relationship between obesity and blood pressure, but they also need to have some rules of action which they can use in the clinical setting, for example simple rules about the steps that should, or should not, be taken to reduce body weight. Similarly, though general practitioners need to know the causes of secondary hypertension, it may be even more important for them to have some simple rules to decide which cases to refer for investigation.

Improving skills

All professionals have skills. They need to be helped to review those they have, and to discover those which need to be improved or are entirely missing.

People whose skills need improvement may not appreciate this, and may not like being told. For example, most professionals think they know how to measure blood pressure because they are already doing it, but they usually don't know that their readings are approximated to the nearest 10mmHg by digit preference, are subject to errors of 10–20mmHg by not using outsize cuffs, or biased around customary diastolic cutting points. They probably will not believe any of these things except through a practical demonstration of their work in a group. The skills needed are not completely new ones but modifications of skills they already have, whose necessity they will learn best through their own experience.

It is also sometimes necessary to help people discard 'skills' that are useless or harmful. For example, routine measurement of blood pressure in all patients over 80 is a skill which should probably be discarded, or the routine recording of both standing and lying pressures without some reason for this, such as concurrent diabetes.

As with the acquisition of knowledge, it is important to help people to:

1 Acquire new skills
2 Adapt and improve existing skills
3 Discard useless or potentially harmful skills.

PUTTING KNOWLEDGE AND SKILLS INTO ACTION

Almost everyone who acquires new knowledge or skills will say and believe they are going to put them into effect, but good intentions are insufficient.

The most effective way of putting skills into action is to review one's work (perhaps by random sampling of records), identify the weak points, set objectives for improvement, and then repeat the review to see whether action has been taken. This is the process of audit.

Knowledge is not static but changes and grows all the time and the number of articles, books and reports on prevention multiply each year. There is no point in trying to keep up with the whole of the literature. One approach is to read the leaders and scan the articles in 3 or 4 of the more important journals, for example the *British Medical Journal, Journal of the Royal College of Practitioners, Lancet*, the *Journal of Advanced Nursing*, and the *Nursing Times*. You might decide to divide these and other journals between your team to form a journal club, meeting once a month, where each member of the club can present a brief review of what they have read, particularly in relation to what might be applied in your own unit. You will soon find that only a small proportion of new material is of practical and lasting importance, and you may find that you are all better able to avoid being brainwashed by the many purveyors of free lunches and persuasive videotapes competing for your credulity.

It is easy to slide into haphazard adoption of new ideas and often transient discoveries. A good approach is to conduct an annual review, not only of your work but of your policies, for example on the advice you give on salt or use of nicotine chewing-gun, in the light of what you have read during the preceding year.

If you are in doubt about reviewing the literature ask the advice of librarians at the local postgraduate centre, the RCGP library at Princes Gate, London, the BMA library at Tavistock Square, London, or the RCN library at Cavendish Square. The RCGP and RCN librarians can supply updated topic bibliographies on virtually any topic in primary care, and this is usually the best first step into the literature.

If a major trial is reported you may find it difficult to interpret the articles on your own; why not convene a meeting at the local postgraduate centre with a local expert and some other primary care workers through your local faculty of the RCGP, your local course organiser for vocational training, or your primary care nurses section of the RCN? Even if you only find 3 or 4 people attend a meeting to discuss a particular topic you will find the debate more fruitful than sitting in your lonely cell trying to sift the wheat from the chaff.

Improving your skills

Three main types of skill need to be improved.

1 Organisational skills
2 Communication skills
3 Clinical skills, for detection and management of risk factors.

DO IT IN PAIRS

Sit down with someone else and identify the skills that you wish to acquire or improve and practise on each other. Beg, borrow or steal a video so that you can see your communication skills in practice. In general, professionals talk too much and don't listen. Practise saying nothing for at least 30 seconds when there is a pause in a discussion. This often allows people time to gather their thoughts and open up a new line of discussion.

Watch someone good. Find someone whose skills you know are good and watch them at work; then ask if they will watch you and give you some tips.

It is hard to assess your own behaviour with individual patients as they are usually too polite to tell you where you are going wrong. If you are the only person they have ever spoken to about cardiovascular disease you are going to be the best one they have ever spoken to, so the consumers are not in a good position to criticise. Nearly all postgraduate centres have video cameras available on loan to record trainee consultations. If you ask you will almost certainly be encouraged to use the same technique to record (with the patients' permission) some of your own encounters. In most but not all cases, doctors and nurses quickly forget the presence of the camera and return to their natural style of consultation, and patients rarely notice the equipment at all, which is much less obtrusive than ordinary optical photography. Looking at your own performance you will recognise most of your mistakes straight away; it is a cardinal rule of such videotaping that no one should be expected to expose their encounters to criticism by other staff unless they want to. If you have no access to a videocamera you can ask a colleague to help you review your practice once a year, to watch you interviewing or to check the way in which you take a history, measure blood pressure, or give advice.

FINDING TRAINING OPPORTUNITIES

As we write in 1986 there are few training opportunities for people interested in prevention, but you may be fortunate in having appropriate training sessions organised locally; or your health authority may have appointed a cardiovascular disease prevention facilitator (see Chapter 19) who may be able to organise the training you need. If not, why not find out if any other practices are in the same position as your own and organise training sessions?

The GP tutor should help with advice on medical content. The nursing officer responsible for district nurse training should be able to give advice on the most appropriate type of training to give to practice nurses, if there is no course or teaching system for practice nurses locally. Local colleges of further education or the business studies' section of the nearest polytechnic may organise training for receptionists and practice managers, and the RCGP is now organising regular short courses on practice management with a big emphasis on prevention and anticipatory care.

One way of doing this is by audit, preferably reviewing the results with the stimulation of an outsider whose opinion the team respects, invited to the audit meeting.

OPEN UNIVERSITY COURSES

Open University course P575 'Coronary heart disease: reducing the risks' is the first study pack in a series of three, which will provide opportunities for all members of primary care teams to study topics relevant to health promotion and health education. Materials will be flexible, divided in modules, comprising (1) an individual study pack requiring about 30 hours of study for self-paced individual work, and (2) a group work pack for three ineractive group sessions. The individual study pack can be used as an entirely free-standing method of learning. Use of the group work pack is optional. It includes an E30 VHS videotape for group discussion and group leaders' notes giving guidance for group activities. All these materials will be available from the OU from January 1987, at an estimated cost of £25–30 for the individual study pack and £125 for the group work pack. (The address to write to is on page 232).

WORKING WITH UNENTHUSIASTIC COLLEAGUES

Though we may assume enthusiasm in our readers, we cannot make the same assumption about your colleagues unless you are working on this book as a group project, all equally fired with enthusiasm for prevention of cardiovascular disease. In most teams one person is more enthusiastic than others but it is important that the whole team becomes committed to prevention, which is too large a challenge to be left to one individual. Unless all your colleagues are committed from the beginning, the idea will always be thought of as 'Donald's little project' and be tolerated rather than supported by other members of the team.

The best approach will depend on the personal experience and attitudes of your colleagues but there are some techniques which can be used to make things easier. The first of these is not to assume that all conservatism is incorrigible. Nearly all doctors and nurses have at some time been excited by and interested in good clinical work, and in most of them this excitement and interest can be rekindled if ideas are presented responsibly and with imagination.

FINDING ENERGY AND TIME

It is uncommon to find professionals who are completely opposed to improving the quality of care provided to their patients. Lack of enthusiasm usually indicates inertia rather than active opposition.

One way to overcome inertia is to emphasise the importance of cardiovascular disease and the scope for prevention, but information by itself is relatively ineffective in changing behaviour. You will have to ensure that the team has time to acquire the skills and knowledge that are necessary and, even more important, to put them into practice. This usually means more staff.

EXTRA STAFF

Only 15% of practices claim their full quota of reimbursable staff and one of the first arguments to put to your colleagues is the need for more. Top priority is usually for a practice nurse but you may need extra secretarial help to cope with the additional work that anticipatory care requires.

YOUR OWN TIME AND ENERGY

Although it is important that the development of prevention is not seen as your pet project, it is equally important that you are able to contribute extra time and extra energy, particularly during the initial phase. The easiest way to do this is for you to reduce, temporarily, some of your other commitments. Try to budget your time so that it is not your family life that suffers.

FIND A TROJAN HORSE

The proverb 'The prophet is without honour in his own country' is well founded. Rather than try to argue the case monotonously yourself you may be able to find an outsider to ask along to a practice meeting, perhaps a local consultant or a team from another health centre who have developed prevention, or a facilitator if your health authority or Family Practitioner Committee has one to assist primary care teams.

Sometimes the Trojan horse can come in the guise of a new trainee. Trainees are effective agents of change, partly because they can put new items on the team's agenda, partly because they are an extra pair of hands to provide the energy and time to get the project going. A move to new premises or the introduction of a computer are other opportunities to push colleagues into action.

Organising training for others

Various training techniques are commonly used, which can be applied to GPs, nurses, and other primary care staff, separately or in combined groups.

CONFERENCES AND SEMINARS

Until recently, national conferences tended to be dialogues between experts arguing about what other people ought to be doing. Actual doers were almost unrepresented, at least on the platform, and argument centred almost entirely on what could or should be done, rather than experience of actually doing it.

This picture is now beginning to change. With its national coronary prevention campaign which was launched in spring 1987, the DHSS is now officially committed to support for a turn towards a mass prevention strategy, though its preferred emphasis is still on personal rather than civic action, and little or nothing has yet been said about the resource and training implications for primary care teams. However, there does seem to be a firm commitment to support national, regional, and area conferences of GPs and practice and community nurses to share experience and develop local tactics.

ACT (Anticipatory Care Teams) is an informal group of primary care nurses and GPs set up in 1986 to bring together primary care teams with an interest in coronary and stroke prevention. They are planning a national conference in York

(1987) and it is hoped that similar conferences will be held every 2 years thereafter, with a newsletter to keep interest going between these events. The current secretary is Dr Theo Schofield at the Medical Centre, Badgers Crescent, Shipston-on-Stour, Warwickshire.

Though much criticised, the conventional conference or seminar held in a postgraduate centre has a part to play in the promotion of prevention. A seminar can:

1 Transfer information
2 Raise enthusiasm
3 Establish or reinforce the identity of a group of people with a common interest in prevention.

Conferences are an opportunity to get experienced, nationally influential speakers to transmit new ideas to a wide audience. The time available for discussion is always too short. Try not to overload your conference with too many speakers; they are by definition big talkers, and if you try to load more than two speakers into one half-day session there won't be enough time to give your own local people a chance to contribute and thus begin to develop as speakers and teachers themselves. Remember that academic experts often lack experience of applying their ideas to the general population in normal field conditions.

Try to include at least one local person as a speaker, presenting local data, perhaps from randomly sampled records. You should have a policy on cadre development, to build up your own local body of postgraduate teachers. Conferences tend to come alive when they deal constructively with the main problems encountered by the audience, and these problems usually relate more to the social structure and human relationships of primary care than to biological problems about lipids or blood pressure.

Conferences are costly, because the travelling and perhaps the accommodation expenses of speakers must be met. Remember that good speakers are never paid for more than an hour or two of the many hours of travelling time involved, and have to work the next day, so if you save money by accommodating them with local GPs or nurses, get them to bed at a reasonable time.

Pharmaceutical companies are often glad to help financially and with the organisation of conferences and will usually accept a remarkably low profile for their products, but you may find yourself in an embarrassing position if your principal message is about changes in behaviour rather than medication.

Otherwise you must rely on early forward planning to obtain Section 63 support from your health authority. Whoever sponsors your conference, you are likely to find unreasonable resistance to the still rather new but immensely effective idea of joint conferences for GPs, nurses, and other primary care staff. It is essential to stand your ground on this, because shared learning of this kind is much more effective than the segregated teaching of the past.

Verbatim written reports of conferences are rarely worth the considerable extra work they impose on the already exhausted conveners, but it may be a good idea to give a couple of people the task of taking notes of the best bits, one to each session, to put together your own press report for a local newsletter. Make sure you have photocopying facilities available to make quick copies of speakers' notes; they can save you a lot of trouble when the speakers have gone and you can't make sense of your own notes.

The main weaknesses of central seminars are that only small numbers can come, and that behaviour seldom changes solely as a result of attending them. These weaknesses can be partially overcome by producing a written report of the seminar and circulating it widely to the target audience, by setting the seminar in the context of a plan of continuing education activity, and above all by insisting that all participants bring real data from their practices, for example, 10 randomly sampled medical records of men aged 35–64, or the recorded data on smoking status of all patients seen the previous day. Use of such real data helps more modest participants to understand that all teams are only at the beginning of serious mass preventive work, and helps to restrain more garrulous participants from running too far ahead of the evidence. It also provides an opportunity for repeating the sampling procedure in the future, to see how much real progress is being made.

SMALL TOWN MEETINGS

By a small town meeting we mean any meeting which brings together more than one primary care team and attempts to achieve the objectives of a large seminar. Although more time-consuming from the point of view of the educators, the organisation of a number of local seminars is often a very effective way of reaching a much larger proportion of the target population than can be reached by central seminars.

It is obviously not possible on all occasions to find speakers of the same quality round the health authority but it is worth while trying to make a simple video or borrow or rent one of the videos listed on page 204 for use at small town meetings.

HEALTH CENTRE AND SURGERY LEARNING

Probably the most effective means of changing behaviour is by organising education activity in the health centre or surgery provided that the activity:

1 Complements central seminars and small town meetings
2 Involves the whole team
3 Relates to the work of the practice, for example by discussing audit of a 10% or 25% random sample of records
4 Allows the team to set objectives
5 Is part of a process of continuing education with follow-up meetings organised to allow the team to measure progress, or the lack of it, and take appropriate action.

Pharmaceutical companies are often glad of any opportunity to reach GPs, and will help with providing educational videotapes and a buffet lunch, which is always popular. These can be useful as an occasional beanfeast for the staff, but it is a mistake to rely on them as the mainstay of your local continuing education. Not only do they naturally include some element of brainwashing in favour of some prescribed drug, but they also tend to be too long, and provide few opportunities for discussion by your own team of their own local experience. Slick presentation and authoritative statements by teaching-hospital consultants may inhibit imaginative discussion. The MSD Foundation tapes are particularly good in presenting learning material informally, in a way that invites discussion and encourages a diversity of views, but they usually need at least two sessions for each tape, with active use of the written material you get with the tapes, at the stop-points indicated.

FURTHER READING AND AUDIOVISUAL AIDS

Clinical epidemiology by David Sackett, Brian Haynes and Peter Tugwell (Boston: Little Brown & Co, 1985) and *Studying a study and testing a test: how to read the medical literature* by Richard Riegelman (same publishers, 1981) provide good guides on how to read articles critically.

There are many practical tips on organisation of conferences and seminars in the *British Medical Journal*'s anthology of articles *How to do it*, published by the BMA in 1979 and available from Tavistock Square, London WC1H 9JR.

The best source of ideas on teaching GPs (which can be adapted to nurses and other members of the team with little difficulty) is *Teaching general practice* by Jack Cormack, Marshal Marinker, and David Morell (London: Kluwer Medical, 1981).

MSD videotapes are available either on loan from your regional adviser on general practice, or can be bought at relatively low cost from the MSD Foundation, Tavistock House North, London WC1H 9JR.

Chapter 19
HELP FROM THE DHSS, HEALTH AUTHORITIES, ETC

Although most of the tasks described in this book are simple they take time and energy, particularly during the development phase. To undertake them practices need extra resources – extra time, extra energy, and extra money – because more work means more staff if one is not to give up even more time which could be better spent with family or friends.

In this chapter we shall describe some of the sources of help that are available for general practitioners focusing particularly on the help that can be provided by staff working for the local health authority.

Health authorities vary from one to another so generalisations have to be made, and read, with caution. One important feature is common to several progressive health authorities; a facilitator.

WHAT IS A FACILITATOR?

A facilitator is someone who helps primary care teams do all the things they want to do to increase the effectiveness of their preventive work. Facilitators are not there simply to do work for the practice, to measure blood pressure or to write to patients for example, they are there to help primary care teams to change the way they work, develop new systems of working, acquire new knowledge and skills, set objectives, and achieve and measure progress. Facilitators help people change who want to change; they do not try to make people change who do not wish to. Tasks commonly carried out by facilitators are:

Acting as 'cross pollinator' of good ideas from practice to practice.

Setting up practice meetings to discuss workload, costs, method of screening, protocols for referral and role of each member of the team.

Offering help with baseline audit of, for example, blood pressure recording.

Helping receptionists and practice managers with methods of identifying patients to be invited and tagging their records.

Providing guidance for practice nurses and general practitioners in screening procedures, e.g. criteria for referral of risk factors to GP and revision of blood pressure measurement technique.

Providing information and 'back-up' service, e.g. suggested drafts of invitation handout and health summary care, sources of free health education literature, height/weight charts as teaching aids.

Encouraging assessment of progress, e.g. by repeat audits or by a logbook (daybook) in a nurse clinic.

Helping the practice draw up a job description for a practice nurse and calculate the costs of her employment.

Organising workshops, seminars and conferences for practice nurses and general practitioners.

What does the facilitator not do?

The most important point to emphasise is that facilitators do not actually assess or counsel individual patients except in the course of staff training. They are not intended simply to supplement the activities of team members, but to complement the work done by the primary care team. The main reasons for this are logistic. If one facilitator is working in a health authority of 300 000 people there will be about 100 000 people in the at-risk age-groups, with about 1200 general practitioners working in 50 primary care teams. Facilitators' jobs will become impossible if they try to help individual patients, when their real task is to improve the health of the whole population at risk. In fact the principal focus of the facilitator's activity is the population of general practitioners and primary care teams within the health authority, not the target population itself.

Second, facilitators are not employed to make primary care teams change their behaviour by bullying or entreating or persuading. They are there to facilitate change, to make it easier, not to impose it. All facilitators in post have found that there are enough practices which want practical help to change the way they work to keep them fully occupied. Their experience is that there is enthusiasm for change in general practice, and that change can be facilitated by people willing to roll their sleeves up and get stuck in alongside the primary care team, but this does not mean that the facilitators do all the work.

A case study

Practice X is, by many criteria, a good practice. Its members are concerned about their patients, are skilled and careful clinicians, and members of the team get on well with one another. But they do not have a systematic approach to detection and management of high blood pressure, in fact they are not particularly well organised at any activity, even claiming money from the family practitioner committee (FPC).

Following the death of a patient from a stroke, one of the partners arranges a lunchtime meeting on stroke prevention and invites the facilitator to tell them about the work other practices are doing to improve the effectiveness of prevention. She emphasises that the main points are:

1 The need to set objectives
2 The need to measure the degree of coverage
3 The need to involve the whole team, particularly the receptionists, secretaries and practice nurses
4 The probable need for additional resources
5 The means of funding additional staff employed by increased uptake of cervical cytology and immunisation
6 The fact that she is there to help the practice resolve these activities.

Enthused by the visit the practice decides to take on a practice nurse, but good intentions are not translated into action. When the facilitator visits again a month later nothing has happened. Having seen the outcome of good intentions in the past, she has a job description in her handbag, and leaves that for the practice to use to recruit someone to work with them.

Three weeks later the job description is still sitting where she left it, much admired and appreciated but not actually translated into an advertisement. The facilitator offers to take the job description and says she knows a couple of nurses who are looking for work and will phone them so that they can make contact with the practice. This offer is gratefully accepted.

The facilitator helps the senior partner arrange interviews and recruit the nurse. To establish a baseline the facilitator helps the practice staff carry out an audit of a 10% random sample of records. She spends time with the receptionists, showing how to identify people at risk, and, by example, shows how to invite people for a 'health check'.

She also spends time with the practice nurse, takes her to see a couple of other nurses working in preventive systems, and convenes a meeting of the practice as a whole to report on the audit findings and asks the practice what objectives they would like to set. She spends several mornings with the practice nurse during the first week of the new system and arranges any specialist training the practice nurse needs. She shows the practice nurse the range of patient education material that is available and provides for the practice nurse the contact points not only for patient education material but also for local Weight Watchers' clubs and Look After Yourself groups. She also helps the practice nurse do a health check on all members of the practice, partly for experience for the nurse but also so that the practice knows what is involved.

For the first week or two the facilitator drops in often to see the receptionists and the practice nurse, helping them sort out the problems that inevitably crop up. Usually such problems can be solved by passing on tips that the facilitator has picked up from other practices that she is visiting. She tells the practice nurse about the practice nurse study day that has been arranged to provide teaching on topics identified by practice nurses as being topics of particular concern and tells the general practitioners over coffee of a plan to have a lunchtime meeting on hypertension management, for two of the doctors have become more anxious to detect high blood pressure because they are puzzled about the part that ACE inhibitors should play in management of high blood pressure.

As the practice develops a new rhythm of working, the facilitator visits less frequently. She keeps in touch and invites the practice to an audit meeting where they can meet a number of other practices who have also carried out an audit and set up a similar system.

WHAT TO DO IF YOU HAVE A FACILITATOR

By June 1987, 30 health authorities in England, Wales and Northern Ireland were employing facilitators. By the time you read this many more should have been appointed. If your health authority employs a facilitator simply phone her up and ask for help.

WHAT TO DO IF YOUR HEALTH AUTHORITY OR FAMILY PRACTITIONER COMMITTEE DOES NOT HAVE A FACILITATOR

The first step is to convince the health authority that general practice can deliver the goods. There is now evidence from a number of places that this is the case but it may require the GPs in the district health authority, regional health authority, and on the family practitioner committee to be fully briefed.

If the health authority has set preventive objectives then general practices locally can identify with them and specify which could be reached more quickly by investing in development of primary care. The most important link is with the community physician, as he or she will be the person who, in most health authorities, has to argue the case for funds.

If the region has set preventive objectives then it may be possible to persuade the region to invest in a facilitator, particularly where the FPC relates to more than one health authority. Regional authorities have a particularly useful function when it comes to bringing about a marriage between a consortium of health authorities and FPC.

WHO CAN BE A FACILITATOR?

Most of the facilitators employed hitherto have come from a nursing or health education background, or a combination of both, but the most important characteristic is their personality.

Facilitators need a combination of charisma to allow them to help practices discuss a potentially sensitive area, namely failure to deliver an adequate service, combined with determination to stick with a primary care team that has said it wishes to change until change is actually achieved. The inertia in some practices can be overcome only by considerable time and energy, not only from the facilitator but also from team members.

A NOTE FOR HEALTH AUTHORITY READERS

This book is primarily for members of primary care teams but it will be read by some people working for health authorities as community physicians and nursing officers, health education officers, or managers.

If health authorities are to provide help for general practitioners they have to appreciate the problems of general practice and the difficulties primary care teams face in delivering services and achieving change. The following points should be borne in mind when considering ways in which closer links with general practice can be developed.

1. General practitioners are busy and very few have much spare time or energy. This applies particularly to general practitioners who are interested in improving their preventive services.
2. As a corollary of this, general practitioners do not need exhortations to change, they need practical help and assistance. General practitioners are assailed by exhortations from all sides to care better for elderly people, think of the problems of adolescents, think of the health hazards of unemployment, improve their cervical cytology coverage, prescribe more carefully, think of people from ethnic minorities, and a whole host of other priorities that rain down upon primary care teams from above. The majority of practitioners and teams are committed to these objectives in theory. What they need is assistance to put the theory into practice.
3. General practitioners should not be expected to suffer financial disadvantage by improving the service they offer.
4. As a corollary of this, the health authority should recognise that general practitioners who participate in service development at district and regional level do so by the good grace of their partners, and health authorities should consider sessional payments for general practitioners who are making regular and sustained contributions to service development.
5. The primary care team works as a team and is confused if community physicians and nursing officers are obviously not working in concert.
6. General practitioners do not simply want to be told what to do by community physicians or consultants. The general practitioner sees a population that is different from the population seen in hospital and topics such as the management of hyperlipidaemia or hypertension have to be approached in a different way when the whole population is considered and approached through primary care.

OTHER HEALTH AUTHORITY RESOURCES

The health authority can also offer other types of assistance through the staff it employs.

Community nurses seconded to work as practice nurses

Some health authorities second community nurses to work as practice nurses. Close links with the relevant nursing officers are obviously important if a preventive service is to be developed, but problems often arise through confusion of authority, particularly over job description and continuity.

Consultant physicians

Although the health service is often depicted as a service composed of two camps in opposition – the curative and the preventive – an increasing number of consultants, particularly in cardiology, are convinced of the benefits of prevention and are willing to lend their support to properly organised preventive work.

Wherever possible it is therefore important to involve consultant cardiologists from an early stage in the development of a preventive programme, as if they are not, and they see it for the first time as a fully completed and costed bid, they may consider it a threat to their own resources. They are obviously also important as a source of advice about issues such as the management of hypertension and hyperlipidaemia.

COMMUNITY PHYSICIANS

In your campaign for support for your practice the community physician can play an important part.

In most health authorities in which facilitators have been appointed the community physician has been centrally involved in developing the preventive programme and winning the resources necessary for employment of facilitators.

As general practitioners become increasingly interested in the population for which they are responsible, as well as in individual patients who consult them, their interests and those of community physicians come closer together – both are interested in population medicine.

Health education units

Few health education units are sufficiently well resourced to have a member of staff concentrating on prevention of cardiovascular disease. Some do not even manage to have one person solely devoted to health education in primary care. Nevertheless, health education units are valuable sources of advice on leaflet design and wording, if a practice wishes to develop its own, and on availability of educational material. The health education officer will have some leaflets and booklets, know some of the others that are available, and be able to suggest who to contact for more detailed information on certain risk factors.

The 'Look After Your Heart' campaign, launched by the Health Education Council and the DHSS in 1986, will result in the production of more educational materials.

Health visitors

The contribution health visitors can make to prevention varies very much depending upon the number available and their existing workload. Obviously the main theme of the work of health visitors is prevention, but in many parts of the country they are so few that they can concentrate only on child health and development. However, even if a health visitor is unable to make a major contribution to the cardiovascular prevention programme she may be a good source of advice on education and behaviour change and steps should be taken to try to involve her at an early stage, while making it clear that it is up to her to decide how much time she will have available for service delivery.

Dieticians

Most health authorities have too few (if any) community dieticians to expect them to be available to run clinics for people who are obese or have hyperlipidaemia. However, dieticians can offer several resources:

1 Knowledge. The community dietician should be aware of current thinking on complex topics such as the relationship between cholesterol intake and blood cholesterol.
2 Patient education material.
3 Educational methods.

Dieticians should be seen primarily as people who can help with staff training and development, rather than as service providers.

Family practitioner committees

The FPC is slowly changing from a body which reacts passively to general practitioners' requests for payment or information, to one which develops primary health care, in association with related health authorities.

At present few FPCs have sufficient staff to be able to fulfil this new role but some are starting to provide training for practice managers and receptionists. Much of the function of the facilitator could well be regarded as the responsibility of the FPC but, at present, FPCs have less flexibility in their budgets than health authorities. Health authorities may as yet provide a more appropriate intellectual base for a facilitator because the other staff employed by health authorities have more similar skills.

However, we shall certainly see FPCs taking a more active part in service development in future. It is important to remind the FPC that the staff it funds have a major contribution to make, not only to disease management but to prevention of cancer, stroke, and heart disease. Because of the substantial lay membership of the committee it is likely that a paper outlining the scope for prevention and the need for support for primary care teams who wish to develop a preventive service would be better received than a similar paper referred to the local medical committee because, in general, the lay public is more enthusiastic about prevention than the medical profession.

Research and public campaigning bodies

All serious innovation in primary care must start with audit, a local study of what is actually going on. Audit is a form of research. Health authorities already at their wits' end to pay for traditional demand-oriented care are generally not enthusiastic about funding the sort of large-scale search for needs implied by this book, and their first instinct is often to solve this problem by describing audited innovation as research, in order to tap alternative sources of funding.

Such suggestions should be resisted. The people on grant-giving bodies are not fools. Plans for service innovation disguised as research will not be accepted, and the attempt may discredit your unit and prejudice later genuine research applications. If your health authority cannot or will not make the staff or other resources available to implement what is fast becoming official DHSS policy, despite your best efforts to rally support on the relevant committees, including the community health council (CHC), and perhaps local press and radio, an honest statement of your plight to one of the national grant-giving bodies may be successful in getting pump-priming money for innovation. If your innovation is successful, you may then be able to persuade your health authority into supporting a second application. The Chest, Heart, and Stroke Association, and the King Edward's Hospital Fund, are two bodies which will give you excellent advice on potential expert support in your area, and may be able to give you some initial help financially. The British Heart Foundation (BHF) is much bigger, richer, and more powerful than either of these, but is heavily oriented towards high-technology hospital care and research. There is pressure on the BHF to pay more attention to primary care and prevention, and a really good research protocol stands a good chance of getting BHF funding, but they are unlikely to support service innovation. Addresses are given on pages 233–4.

SOURCES OF HELP AND ADVICE

The Oxford Prevention of Heart Attack and Stroke Project, funded by the Health Education Authority, Oxfordshire Health Authority and the Chest, Heart and Stroke Association is able to help Health Authorities and Family Practitioner Committees find, recruit and train facilitators. Contact Claire Fullard, Project Director, at the Radcliffe Infirmary, Woodstock Road, Oxford OX2 6HE.

Chapter 20
EDUCATIONAL LEAFLETS

In various chapters we have mentioned the desirability of having leaflets available to hand out to patients. We offer the following four as suggested material. It is for you, the reader, to take and use them in any adapted form which is suitable for your local needs. The topics covered are high blood pressure, non-insulin-dependent diabetes, weight-reducing, cholesterol-lowering diet and low sodium, low fat diet.

What you need to know about high blood pressure

Everyone has a blood pressure (BP), without it their blood would not circulate. The higher your BP is, the greater your risk of coronary heart disease, heart failure, stroke, retinal bleeding or detachment, and kidney failure, particularly if you also smoke or have diabetes. High BP is not a disease, but a treatable cause of these serious diseases. Unless it has already caused one of them, high BP seldom causes symptoms. It can be very high indeed without causing headaches, breathlessness, palpitations, faintness, giddiness, or any of the other symptoms traditionally thought to be caused by high BP, and you may have any or all of these symptoms without having high BP. The only way to tell what your BP is, is to measure it with a BP manometer.

MECHANISMS

The level of BP depends on how hard your heart pumps blood into your arteries, on the total volume of blood in your circulation, and on how tight your arteries are. The smaller arteries are sheathed by a spiral muscle, which makes them wider or narrower according to the needs of the body. In people with high BP something goes wrong with this mechanism, so that the arteries are too tight, and the heart has to beat harder to push blood through them. This tightening-up can occur as a result of nervous or chemical signals, chiefly from the brain, the larger arteries, and the kidneys.

CAUSES

The causes of transient rises in BP are well understood, but these are not what we mean by high blood pressure. High blood pressure is important only when it is sustained for many years; it is high average pressure which is important, not occasional peaks. The causes of such long-term rises in pressure are not fully known, though we do know that high BP runs strongly in families.

High BP is also caused by overweight, particularly in young people. If you have a fat upper arm (more than 30 centimetres (12 inches) circumference), BP cannot be measured accurately without an outsize cuff for the manometer; many doctors, both GPs and in hospitals, don't have outsize cuffs, and if they use a standard cuff on a fat arm they may record false high pressures and start you on treatment you don't really need. However, even with an outsize cuff, overweight is an important cause of high BP and weight reduction is a sensible first step in treating it.

Weight loss depends mainly on eating less fat, meat, sugar and alcohol and more fruit, vegetables, cereal foods and fish. Some of these foods have other beneficial effects as well as helping weight loss. There is good evidence that eating less fat and limiting alcohol to not more than 4 drinks (glasses of wine, single measures of spirits, or half-pints of beer) a day reduces BP, apart from any effect on weight. These changes in diet will also reduce risk of coronary heart disease by lowering blood cholesterol. Heavy drinking (more than 8 drinks a day) is a common and important cause of high BP which is often overlooked.

Stress

BP rises for a few minutes or hours if you are anxious, angry, have been hurrying, have a full bladder, or if you are cold, so BP measured at such times is not reliable, but none of these things seems to be a cause of permanently raised BP. High BP seems to be almost as common in peaceable, even-tempered people without worries, as it is in excitable people with a short fuse.

The evidence on this is conflicting, and feeling pushed at work or at home may be an important cause in many people, but this is certainly not true for everyone. It is important to understand that the word 'hypertension', which in medical jargon has exactly the same meaning as 'high blood pressure', does not mean that feeling tense necessarily raises BP, nor does it mean that everyone with a high BP feels tense. Training in relaxation certainly lowers BP for a while (BP falls profoundly during normal sleep), and probably has a useful long-term effect on high BP in people who learn how to 'switch off' frequently during the day. There is no evidence that treatment by relaxation is an effective or safe alternative to drug treatment in people with severe high BP.

Salt

The usual British diet contains far more salt than anyone needs, and it does no harm to reduce intake by not adding salt to cooked meals, by avoiding high-salt processed foods (sausages, sauces, tinned meats and beans, and canned foods generally), Chinese take-aways (which contain huge quantities of sodium glutamate), and strong cheeses. Milk and bread contain surprisingly large amounts of salt.

There is no convincing evidence that the roughly one-third reduction in salt intake you can achieve by these changes in diet will reduce moderately raised BP, or that salt restriction of this degree is a safe or effective alternative to drug treatment for severe high BP. However, people with BP high enough to need drugs can usually manage on a lower dose if they reduce salt intake, and very heavy salt-eaters should certainly try to cut down. There is much better evidence that reducing fat in your diet reduces BP, as well as reducing blood cholesterol, and you may find it difficult to reduce fat and salt at the same time.

Smoking

Smoking is not a cause of high BP, but if you have high BP already, your risk of a heart attack is doubled by smoking over age 50, even more at younger ages; heart attacks in people under 45 occur almost entirely in smokers. Smoking is a very powerful risk factor in its own right, not only for coronary heart disease, but also for cancer of the lung, bladder, and pancreas, and for chronic obstructive lung disease. People who take the trouble to treat their high BP with pills but continue to smoke need their heads tested.

WHEN SHOULD HIGH BLOOD PRESSURE BE TREATED WITH DRUGS?

High blood pressure should be treated with drugs if there is already evidence of damage to the brain, heart, eyes or kidneys, and in all diabetics. Otherwise it should be treated only if the average BP (calculated from at least 3 readings on separate days) is at or over about 175/105 (you don't need to know what these figures mean, but you should know what, in your own case, they are, just as you should know your own height and weight). This threshold (or something like it, plus or minus 5 either way) is derived from the evidence of several big, controlled trials in Britain, Australia, and the USA, which have shown worthwhile saving of life in treated as against untreated cases. Most of the benefit has been in reduced strokes, heart failure, and kidney damage; the effects on coronary heart attacks have been generally unconvincing.

DRUGS FOR HIGH BLOOD PRESSURE

The aim of all treatment of high BP is not cure (the tendency to high BP usually lasts all your life) but prevention. People with severe high BP are likely to live longer if their BP is reduced by drugs, than if they are left untreated, but they seldom feel better and often feel worse.

People with BP averaging 175/105 or more nearly always need drugs to control it, which usually have to be continued for the rest of their lives. All drugs used for high BP cause unpleasant side-effects in some people, though the newer drugs are generally much easier to take than the older ones. If you think your drugs are upsetting you, say so; there are many alternative treatments.

Failure of erection is quite a common side-effect of several drugs in common use, and if this happens make sure you tell the doctor about it; it will clear up soon after your drugs are changed. Other common side-effects are tiredness, depression, and shortness of breath or wheezing. Don't try to alter your medication yourself.

FOLLOW-UP

Always bring your tablets with you when you see the doctor or nurse for follow-up, so that both of you know exactly which drugs you are talking about. If your BP refuses to fall despite apparently adequate medication, think about your weight, your salt intake, or alcohol. Follow-up visits will be frequent at first, perhaps once a week, until your BP is controlled to about 160/90 or less. After that most doctors like to check BP every 3 months or so; never go longer than 6 months without a check.

What you need to know about non-insulin-dependent diabetes

Diabetes is a condition in which there is too much glucose in the blood. Insulin is a hormone, a chemical produced in the pancreas, which controls the level of blood glucose. There are two kinds of diabetes: insulin-dependent diabetes (ID), which mainly begins in youth, is seldom inherited, and requires insulin injections to maintain life; and non-insulin-dependent diabetes (NID), which runs strongly in families, usually starts in middle or old age, and in which the level of blood glucose can be controlled by diet alone, or by diet plus blood glucose lowering tablets. More than twice as many people have NID as ID.

The main cause of NID is an inherited tendency to store energy as fat, together with taking in more energy from your food than you can use up. It therefore happens almost entirely in people who are overweight, and by far the most important part of treatment is to change your eating habits to a more suitable diet.

People with large reserves of energy stored as fat need more insulin from their own pancreas. As they get older this organ gets worn out, unable to produce as much insulin as they need to maintain their excess fat; they become insulin deficient, their body cells become unable to use glucose efficiently, and unused glucose piles up in their blood, eventually overflowing into urine. If you can overcome the obesity, you can in two-thirds of all cases cure the diabetes without antidiabetic tablets. These drugs work by increasing output of insulin from the worn-out pancreas, and for many people with NID they are necessary, but the first step for *every* diabetic is to stick closely to a suitable diet which reduces energy input, and the second step is to try to take more exercise so that more energy taken is used, and not stored as fat.

What happens if you don't? Sustained high blood glucose has two main effects: an immediate effect by spilling over the normal barrier to glucose in the kidney so that glucose appears in the urine, and a long-term effect on arteries supplying blood to all organs in your body. Glucose in urine allows germs to grow which cause infection in the bladder and kidneys, and yeasts to grow on the skin around the penis and vagina (thrush); attacks of bladder trouble and itchy rashes are a warning that diabetes is out of control.

The long-term effect on arteries is much more serious: high blood glucose goes together with high blood cholesterol, laying down a waxy substance in the walls of the arteries (atheroma) which obstructs the flow of blood. Obstruction of large leg arteries may cause pain in the calves or buttocks, obstruction of the coronary arteries may cause pain across the front of the chest on walking (angina) or heart attacks, and obstruction of arteries in the neck may cause transient or permanent brain damage (stroke). Obstruction of the smallest arteries all over the body may cause severe damage to the retina of the eye with loss of useful vision (though complete blindness is rare), to the kidney causing kidney failure, to the nerves controlling sex function causing impotence, and to nerves supplying sensation to the legs and feet. The combination of nerve damage and poor circulation of blood in the feet makes them particularly vulnerable, and good foot care is essential for all diabetics.

All these effects can be prevented by good control of your diabetes: conscientious dieting, more exercise, regular tablets if you need them, and a regular medical check once or twice a year for warning signs of any of these complications, most of which are treatable at an early stage.

A weight-reducing, cholesterol-lowering diet sheet

This diet is suitable for diabetics, people with high blood pressure or high blood cholesterol, and for anyone who wants to reach a healthier weight.

There are six golden rules:

Eat less high-energy food
Stop nibbling between meals
Take more exercise
Eat less fat
Eat more vegetables, fruit, and cereals
Measure what you have achieved honestly and regularly.

REDUCE ENERGY INTAKE

Your body needs fuel to work, as well as other kinds of food for maintenance and repairs. The fuel part of your food we call energy (measured in calories), and that is the sense in which we use the word here. Don't let the advertisers kid you that you need to eat more energy to feel less tired; you would probably feel a lot more energetic if you were eating less energy!

Reducing energy intake means eating less, partly by avoiding between-meal nibbles and snacks, and partly by selectively reducing intake of high-energy foods, particularly sugars (don't forget pop and glucose drinks), fats, and alcohol. Proof that this is actually happening is a slow but steady fall in weight to a target which should be negotiated individually for each patient. Losing a few pounds over the first couple of weeks is usually fairly easy, but the more important aim is a small steady loss of perhaps 1lb+ a week over many months, to achieve target weight and stay there. Your new diet is for life, not a gimmick for a quick blitz and then pile it all on again.

INCREASE ENERGY THROUGHPUT

Diabetics achieve better control and reduce their coronary risks if they use more energy by taking regular exercise, even if the balance between food input and exercise output remains the same.

REDUCE FAT INTAKE

Fat (which includes oil, cream, and the concealed fat of cheeses, chocolate, and all fried foods) is not only an extremely concentrated form of energy, but also the main source of blood cholesterol, which is the main cause of atheroma in the coronary arteries, aorta, neck and thigh arteries. Though cholesterol in foods is not good for you, most body cholesterol is made from other fats; what we aim for is not so much a low-cholesterol diet, as a diet that does not generate cholesterol. Some fats raise cholesterol much more than others. In general, fats from farmed animals (saturated fats), both as fat on and in meat, and as milk, cream, butter, hard margarines, and cheese are big cholesterol-raisers. Most vegetable fats and fish oils (polyunsaturated fats) tend to lower blood cholesterol. They are contained in corn and sunflower oil, in most soft margarines, and in mackerel, herring, trout and salmon. Processed foods often contain large amounts of fat which are not at all obvious: sausages are often about 50% fat.

There is also good evidence that reducing fat in diet lowers blood pressure.

In most working-class diets, the biggest source of fat is frying in general, and chips in particular. The aim should be to reduce fat to about 25% of total energy intake; that is, to reduce the present average intake by about one-third. You can do this by drinking semi-skim milk (which, unlike skimmed milk, you can adapt to very quickly), by eating less and leaner meat, by grilling, steaming, or micro-waving rather than frying, and by not automatically spreading butter or margarine on every slice of bread.

EAT MORE FIBRE: VEGETABLES, FRUIT, AND CEREALS

Plant foods have two big virtues: they don't contain animal fats, so they don't promote blood cholesterol, and they contain large quantities of indigestible residues, commonly called 'fibre'. In fact, as well as fibrous material derived from the cellulose walls of plant cells, they include various gums which are not fibrous at all.

The positive effects of these residues are:

to slow down the absorption of food from the gut, so that the pancreas does not have to produce so much insulin quickly: this is important for diabetics;

to make eating harder work – you have to chew more for each unit of energy taken, so over-eating is more difficult;

to improve gut function, preventing constipation and piles, gallstones, diverticulitis, and probably reducing risk of bowel cancer.

Very large amounts of added fibre, usually bran, can cause quite severe colic and even intestinal obstruction in obsessional dieters who rush into new diets. Plant foods in general, and pulses (beans, peas, and lentils) in particular, produce a lot of gas during fermentation in the gut, and this has to go somewhere. This seems to be less of a problem once your gut gets used to a more vegetarian diet, and the answers are to start slowly, and not to overdo it. As well as bran, you can add 'fibre' to your diet by using one of the prescribable preparations of guar gum, which often improve control of diabetes.

A low sodium, low fat diet for poorly controlled high blood pressure

When high blood pressure is difficult to control, a big reduction in salt intake may bring it down. This is specially true of patients treated with ACE inhibitor drugs (captopril and enalapril), which are used only for difficult cases, and may not be effective unless salt intake is restricted. A low fat diet is essential for all people with high blood pressure, whether it is easy or difficult to control, because all are otherwise at high risk of premature hardening of the arteries. There is also good evidence that a reduction in dietary fat reduces blood pressure. Low-sodium diets tend to taste rather uninteresting, particularly during the first two or three months, and unless a conscious effort is made to reduce fat intake, you may find yourself eating a more fatty diet in an attempt to make dull food more tasty. The evidence against fat is better than the evidence against salt, so if you can't cope with both, cut down on fat rather than salt.

Salt is composed of two elements, sodium and chlorine. It is the sodium which matters for blood pressure, whether or not it is combined with chlorine as ordinary table salt.

MEASURING YOUR SODIUM INTAKE

Sodium intake is measured in millimols (mmol). The easiest way to measure daily intake is not to analyse your food, but to measure sodium output, which except in very hot weather is almost entirely in urine, and should be the same as intake. This is done by collecting *all* the urine passed during 7 days, measuring the volume of urine each day in millilitres (ml), and keeping a small sample from each day's collection for laboratory analysis at the end of the week. (The exact procedure is given at the end of this leaflet (p. 229).) It looks very complicated at first sight, but compared with the difficulties of reducing sodium intake, it's easy. The results will help you to comply with the diet, and you will find the effort well worth while.

Why do we need to measure sodium intake over 7 days? Why isn't one day enough? The aim is to estimate how much sodium you normally eat and drink on average. Many studies have shown that the amount of sodium people take varies enormously from one day to the next, and measurements based on one day only are likely to be misleading. Average daily intakes in this country are usually around 180mmol in men and 150mmol in women, but individuals may vary from about 110mmol a day to 350mmol or more; obviously you need to know where you are starting from.

Having measured your intake before starting a low-sodium diet, this procedure should be repeated 3 or 4 months after going on the diet. Only in this way will you know how successful you have been. People who guess how much sodium they are eating are nearly always wrong. In our experience reduction of sodium is difficult for most patients, and you will find it much easier if you have some good evidence that you are achieving something by your efforts.

ACHIEVING YOUR TARGET

If the second measurement shows a daily intake below 100mmol for an average man, or 80mmol for an average woman, you are doing all right. How can this be achieved?

Obviously the first thing you will do is to stop adding any salt to your food after it's cooked, and avoid very salty foods like kippers, but obviously salty foods are not the main sources of sodium in most people's diet. Monosodium glutamate is added to many processed foods to improve flavour, bringing Chinese take-away meals to high sodium loads of 200mmol or more per portion. Generally speaking, off-the-shelf prepared convenience foods tend to contain much more sodium than home-cooked foods. Sodium nitrite is a commonly-added preservative, and because the entire food industry is competing for instant flavour-appeal, processed foods are now the main (and not always obvious) source of dietary sodium. For example, one average-sized potato contains 0.2mmol sodium compared with 21mmol in one cupful of instant mashed potato; one portion of Kentucky Fried Chicken contains 75mmol, and one portion of branded hamburger and chips contains 97mmol. Some cough medicines also contain high amounts of sodium; as cough medicines are usually ineffective, the best thing is not to take them. About one-third of dietary sodium usually comes from bread, and one of the first things you will have to do is to find a local source of low-sodium bread or flour. As the sodium content of bread cannot be reduced much below half without making it impossible to bake, even then you will have to limit your bread intake.

THREE RULES FOR A LOW SODIUM, LOW FAT DIET

If you follow these 3 rules, you should be able to achieve your target. Make your changes slowly, dropping off the forbidden foods one at a time, allowing 3 or 4 months before you reach your target. You will find that gradually your taste changes, so that foods you once thought to be not very salty, now taste too salty.

STOP these very salty or fatty foods, which should be avoided altogether:

SAUCES and CONDIMENTS: Bovril, Marmite, Oxo, chutneys and bottled sauces, laverbread.
SMOKED and TINNED FISH: kippers and bucklings, smoked

haddock, cockles, mussels, prawns and shrimps, scampi, tinned salmon, sardines and pilchards.

MOST BREAKFAST CEREALS: Weetabix, All Bran, Rice Krispies, cornflakes, Special K, Frosties.

SNACKS: salted nuts, pork scratchings, pork pies, pasties.

MOST MILK PRODUCTS and CHEESE: evaporated or condensed milk, tinned cream, all hard, soft, or processed cheese other than cottage cheese, salted butter or margarine.

MOST SOUPS: canned and packet soups. Though you can cook your own soups with little or no salt, most people find these inedible.

SAVOURY BISCUITS and PASTRY: crispbreads, cheese biscuits, cocktail biscuits, self-raising flour, cornflour, baking powder, frozen or packet pastry.

PRESERVED MEATS: sausages, fried or boiled bacon, fried or cooked ham, tongue, jellied veal, luncheon meat.

CANNED VEGETABLES, BAKED BEANS and TOMATOES.

DRIED FRUITS.

GOLDEN SYRUP, CHOCOLATE, TOFFEES.

ORDINARY BROWN, WHITE or WHOLEMEAL BREAD.

NEVER use sodium bicarbonate when cooking vegetables.

THINK about the following salty foods, which you may allow yourself in small amounts:

PORRIDGE, Ready Brek, muesli, Alpen, prunes.

MILK: not more than half a pint a day, yoghourt, ice cream, cream and cottage cheese.

CURRIES.

UNSALTED FISH.

LOW-SALT BREAD, preferably wholemeal.

EGGS: unsalted eggs don't contain much sodium, but are high in fat and cholesterol. You can allow yourself 2 a week.

UNSALTED BUTTER or Flora and similar polyunsaturated margarines.

UNSALTED NUTS.

GO AHEAD and eat as much as you like of the following low-sodium foods. You can liven them up with vinegar, mint and other herbs, spices, mustard, home-made salad dressings, pepper, and lemon juice.

Shredded Wheat, Sugar Puffs.

ALL FRESH FRUITS, ALL FRESH or HOME-COOKED VEGETABLES, RICE, FRESH MEAT, FISH and POULTRY, SPAGHETTI and MACARONI.

PROCEDURE FOR COLLECTING 24-HOUR URINE

Each day's collection begins with the *second* lot of urine passed after waking, and ends with the *first* lot of urine passed the next day. On DAY 1 the first lot should be passed into the toilet as usual. *All* urine passed during the next 24 hours should be passed into the large container provided, which is marked along the side in millilitres (ml). After the first day's collection is complete, read off the total volume of urine in ml and write down the figure. Then pour a little of the urine into one of the small plastic containers. Then pour away the rest of the urine and start the next day's collection, and so on until you have done 7 days, with 7 small containers full of urine and 7 measurements of the total amount of urine in ml. If you keep these in a cool place they can all be sent to the laboratory at once when the collection is finished.

Leave your big container in the toilet you normally use. You will need another smaller container for use when you are away from home, which you can empty into the big container. You will be supplied with some disinfectant, which you should add to each container before you start collecting each day to avoid smells. Be careful with it, it will hurt your skin if it comes into contact.

Remember to empty your bladder first, before you open your bowels. Some people find this easier to remember if they fix a safety pin across their underwear.

You are bound to forget occasionally, and pass some or all of your urine into the toilet. If this happens, estimate the amount you have lost, write it down, and let us know about it when you return your containers to the surgery.

USEFUL ADDRESSES

HEALTH EDUCATION AND FURTHER EDUCATION FOR THE TEAM

Health Education Council, 78 New Oxford St, London WC1A 1AH
01–637 1881

Scottish Health Education Unit, 21 Lansdowne Crescent, Edinburgh EH12 5EH
031–337 3251

Open University Department of Health and Social Welfare, Walton Hall, Milton Keynes MK7 6AA
0908–653743

Your Health Authority, listed in the local phone directory, will have a Health Education Officer.

Names and addresses of Regional Advisers in general practice, Course Organisers and General Practice Tutors are given each year in the RCGP Members' Reference Book.

If you plan to use local or regional newsmedia, Denis MacShane's book *Using the Media* (Pluto Press, London, 1979) is very helpful, and contains regional lists of useful addresses.

SMOKING

Action on Smoking and Health (ASH), 27–35 Mortimer St, London W1N 7RJ
01–637 9843
This is the main campaigning organisation

Dr Chris Steele (expert on use of nicotine chewing-gum) 14 Belfield Rd, Didsbury, Manchester M20 0BH

Lundbeck Laboratories Ltd (manufacturers of nicotine chewing-gum), Lundbeck House, Hastings Street, Luton, Bedforshire LU1 5BE

PROFESSIONAL AND SPECIAL INTEREST ORGANISATIONS

Look through this list for ideas about organisations which may be able to help you with advice, putting you in touch with the right experts and practical innovators, or even occasionally with a little initial funding.

Anticipatory Care Teams (ACT), c/o Dr Theo Schofield, The Medical Centre, Badgers Crescent, Shipston-on-Stour, Warwickshire CV36 4BD
This recently formed group brings together doctors, nurses, and other primary health workers with an interest in coronary and stroke prevention programmes

Association for the Study of Obesity, c/o Margaret Ashwell, MRC Dunn Nutrition Unit, Milton Road, Cambridge CB4 1XJ

Association of Community Health Councils for England & Wales (*sec*: M.A.Gerrard,) 362 Euston Road, London NW1 3BL

British Cardiac Society (*sec*: Mrs G. Read) 2 Beaumont Street, London W1H 2DX

British Diabetic Association, 10 Queen Anne Street, London W1M 0BD

British Heart Foundation, 102 Gloucester Place, London W1H 4DH

British Medical Association, Tavistock Square, London WC1H 9JP

Chest, Heart, and Stroke Association, Tavistock House North, Tavistock Square, London WC1H 9JE

Confederation of Health Service Employees, Glen House, High Street, Banstead, Surrey SM7 2LH

Coronary Prevention Group (*director*: Anne Dillon) Central Middlesex Hospital, London NW10 7NS 01–961 6993 ext.2330
This has been the principal campaigning group on coronary prevention, with very wide contacts, and able to provide reliable data on every aspect of coronary disease prevention

Council for Postgraduate Medical Education in England & Wales, 7 Marylebone Road, London NW1 5HH

Council on Epidemiology and Prevention of the International Society and Federation of Cardiology (*sec*: Dr Peter Schnohr) Romesgade 3, 1362 Copenhagen-K, Denmark.
This is the principal international clearing house for information on research and innovation in coronary and stroke prevention at primary care level through the *CVD Newsletter* (ed. Dr Fred Epstein) Lindenstrasse 31, 8008 Zurich, Switzerland. New members are welcomed

Edinburgh Postgraduate Board for Medicine, Pfizer Foundation, Hill Square, Edinburgh EH8 9DR

Faculty of Community Medicine of the Royal Colleges of Physicians of the United Kingdom, 28 Portland Place, London W1N 4DE

Health Visitors Association, 36 Eccleston Square, London SW1V 1PF

Heartbeat Wales (*director*: Professor John Catford) Ty George Thomas, 24 Park Place, Cardiff CF1 3BA

King Edward's Hospital Fund for London, 14 Palace Court, London W2 4HT
The Fund has always promoted service innovation, and is a good source of literature and information on pioneering projects of all kinds. It maintains an information centre with good conference facilities at the King's Fund Centre, 126 Albert Street, London NW1 7NF

Medical Council on Alcoholism, 31 Bedford Square, London WC1B 3JS

MSD Foundation, Tavistock House, Tavistock Square, London WC1H 9LG (for training videotapes)

National Union of Public Employees, Civic House, 20 Grand Depot Road, Woolwich, London SE18 6SF

Northern Ireland Council for Postgraduate Medical Education, 5 Annadale Avenue, Belfast BT7 3JH

Nutrition Society, Chandos House, Queen Anne Street, London W1M 9LE

Office of Population Censuses and Surveys, St Catherine's House, 10 Kingsway, London WC2B 6JP

This is what used to be the Registrar General's Office. They can be very helpful in providing local mortality statistics, either on standard local authority boundaries or using areas defined by any combination of postcodes

Oxford Prevention of Heart Attack and Stroke project: they can give advice and practical help to health authorities who wish to employ a facilitator. Contact Community Health Offices, Radcliffe Infirmary, Oxford OX2 6HE

Royal College of General Practitioners, 14 Princes Gate, London SW7 1PU

Royal College of Nursing, 20 Cavendish Square, London W1M 0AB

Royal College of Physicians, 11 St Andrew's Place, London NW1 4LE

Royal College of Physicians of Edinburgh, 9 Queen Street, Edinburgh EH2 1JQ

Royal College of Physicians and Surgeons of Glasgow, 234 St Vincent Street, Glasgow G2 5RJ

Royal Society of Health, 38A St George's Drive, London SW1V 3QN

Scottish Council for Postgraduate Medical Education, 8 Queen Street, Edinburgh EH2 1JE

INDEX

Note: Page references in *italic* are locations for figures in text